African-Caribbean Hairdressing

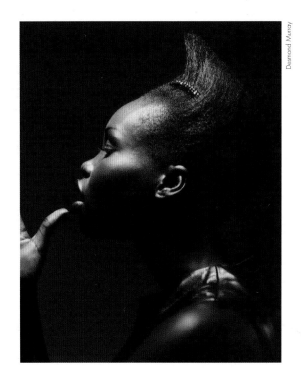

Desmond Murray

African-Caribbean Hairdressing

Sandra Gittens

with contributions from Car-ron Grazette,
Patricia Livingston and Karlene Morrison-Briscoe

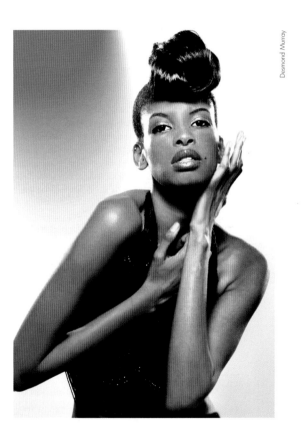

Desmond Murray

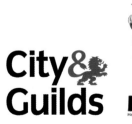
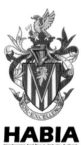

City&Guilds   HABIA   THOMSON

Hairdressing And Beauty Industry Authority

Australia · Canada · Mexico · Singapore · Spain · United Kingdom · United States

THOMSON

African-Caribbean Hairdressing – 2nd Edition

Copyright © Sandra Gittens, Car-ron Grazette, Patricia Livingston and Karlene Morrison-Briscoe 2002

The Thomson logo is a registered trademark used herein under licence.

For more information, contact Thomson Learning, High Holborn House, 50-51 Bedford Row, London WC1R 4LR or visit us on the World Wide Web at: http://www.thomsonlearning.co.uk

British Library Cataloguing-in-Publication Data
A catalogue record for this book is available from the British Library

ISBN-13: 978-1-86152-804-3
ISBN-10: 1-86152-804-3

First edition published in 1988 by Macmillan Press Ltd
Reprinted 2001 by Thomson Learning
Second edition published in 2002 by Thomson Learning
Reprinted 2003 and 2005 by Thomson Learning

Typeset by Tek-Art, Croydon, Surrey

Printed and bound in Italy by G. Canale & C.

Note about pronouns
Using "he or she" and "him and her" throughout the text would become cumbersome in a book such as this. For simplicity and ease of reading therefore, we have generally used simply "she" and "her", except in passages specifically concerned with men's hairdressing.

This book is dedicated to my mother and written in memory of my father.
To my mother Beryl Gittens, thank you for your inspiration, guidance and tuition
throughout the years. The knowledge you shared, is the foundation of this book.

Contents

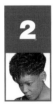

3 Shampooing and conditioning 31

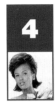
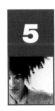
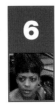

7

Chemical relaxing 93

8

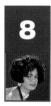

Perming 117

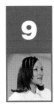

Thermal styling 137

Cutting 151

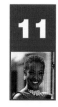

Colouring 177

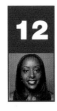
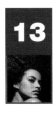

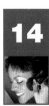

14 Black skin care and make-up 277

15 Health and safety 297

Foreword

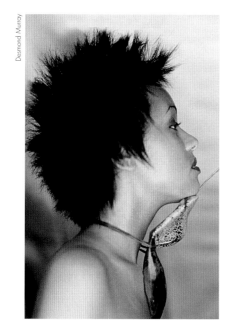

This is the second edition of the much loved and respected book from Sandra Gittens. Since 1988, when the first edition was published, the world of hairdressing has changed greatly and this book reflects those changes.

My foreword for the first edition talked about the veritable cornucopia of information that can be gleaned from Sandra. This new edition, again with support from Car-ron Grazette, Patricia Livingston and Karlene Morrison, has reached new heights and pushes the art of African-Caribbean hairdressing into the forefront of the public eye.

Fast becoming the essential book for African-Caribbean hairdressers throughout the world, I'm delighted to be writing this foreword. If your desire is to excel in the ever changing world of African-Caribbean Hairdressing, then reading this book should be your first step.

Alan Goldsbro
Chief Executive Officer
Hairdressing And Beauty Industry Authority

Preface

When the mainstay of your profession calls for the correct
knowledge, guidelines and techniques for working with
African-Caribbean hair, you need look no further, as we
now have a very comprehensive and informative guide on
the subject. Time, next to talent, is your most valuable
resource.

The test of effective educational material is how well it can
be used for maximum efficiency in learning. Make time for
this book as it will help you beat the clock. Every stylist
who aspires to becoming accomplished in African-Caribbean
hairdressing will benefit from reading it.

Winston Isaacs

The author

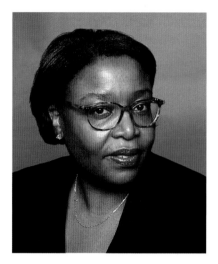

Sandra Gittens grew up in a hairdressing environment, her mother having opened one of the earlier African-Caribbean hairstyling salons in the mid 1960s in Streatham. She has worked in the industry for over 20 years both as a hairdresser and trainer. Her initial training was in Caucasian hairstyling techniques and beauty therapy. In the early 1970s her parents decided to return to Guyana in South America, to establish their individual businesses. Her mother and herself opened a hairdressing salon in Georgetown, the capital of Guyana. It was here that Sandra, under the guidance and tuition of her mother Beryl Gittens, developed her knowledge of the specialist skills of African-Caribbean hairstyling techniques. Guyana's multicultural environment enabled Sandra to develop skills across a wide range of hair types.

In November 1981 Sandra returned to England with the intention of studying trichology, but instead launched herself into a career lecturing in hairdressing. Her first educational post was at City and East London College. In 1986 she joined the London College of Fashion as a lecturer; whilst teaching here she studied for her Certificate in Education. Sandra is currently Course Director for the Image Styling Hair and Make-up course at the college. She has a BA Honours in Education. She has also been chair of Specialist Hair and Beauty associates and acted as a consultant for HABIA and several other training organisations. Her links with industry mean that she is constantly asked to judge competitions and sits on a number of committees in an advisory capacity.

In 1997 Sandra was awarded the Black Heritage Industry Award by Luster Products for her contributions to the hairdressing industry.

Notes on the contributors

Car-ron Grazette trained at the London College of Fashion and is a trichologist and a hairdresser. She has taught hairdressing in further education, and currently runs a busy London salon. She is also a technician for Luster Products (Europe), and presents many shows for them both in the UK and overseas.

Contributing chapters: Hair Characteristics; and Health and Safety.

Patricia Livingston grew up in a hairdressing environment, and currently runs and manages a family hairdressing business. She has worked as a technician and acts as a consultant and trainer for Goldwell (Hair Cosmetics) Ltd. She is also a part-time lecturer at the London College of Fashion.

Contributing chapters: Colouring; Hair Extensions; and Natural Hair. Curlise Dixon contributed the laser weave section in the Hair Extensions chapter.

Karlene Morrison-Briscoe is a qualified beauty therapist with a successful mobile business. She also teaches at Lambeth College, London. She trained at the London College of Fashion.

Contributing chapter: Black Skin Care and Make-up.

Acknowledgements

The author and publishers would like to thank the following for their contributions to the book:

Angelique Ferron
Angel Ramsey
Anne Braithwaithe
Aubrey and Wesley Gittens
Beauty of the Nile Hair Salon
Brenda Gittens
Burnett Forbes Hair Salon
Car-ron Grazette
Chantae's Salon
Christine Lucien
Chubb Fire Ltd
Claire de Graft
Claudette Burnett
Claudette Thornton
Curlise Dixon
Dawn Gittens
Debra Daley
Depilex
Derrick Mullings
Desmond Murray
Dr A L Wright
Dr M H Beck
Edward and Lyn Murray
Ellisons
Freddie Luster II – Luster
   Products
Gill and Richelle Case
Glenda and Rick Clarke
Glenda Clarke
Goldwell [hair cosmetics] Ltd
Heulwen Jenkins

Ike Mantaf
Ingrid Gittens
Institute of Trichologists
Jennifer Taylor
Jessica Yangtze Nyatedzy
Julette Burnett
June Forbes
Karen Barnett
Karlene Morrison-Briscoe
Kathryn Longmuir at Ishoka
Kizure Ltd
Le Noir Salon
London College of Fashion
   for the use of hair studios
Luster Products (Europe)/
   ArtEffex Salon Systeme/
   Designer Touch
Maddisons Hair and Beauty
Maureen Massay Alstrom
Media Image
Melissa McCullock
Michelle McIntosh
Montaz
New Hibiscus Hair Salon
Nigel Tribbeck for step-by-step
   photography
Parres
Patricia Livingston
Patrick Jacobs
Portia Lewis
Redken

Renbow International
Sam and Rod Kirwan
Serena Newland
Shaz
Sorisa
St Thomas' Hospital

Syd Shelton
Terry Jacques Salon
Vinetta McIntosh
Wella
Winston Isaacs

Thank you to the Murray and Gittens families, who have been a source of encouragement and motivation during the development of both editions of this book.

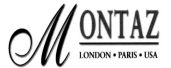

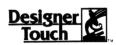

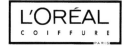

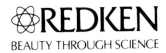
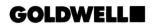

Introduction

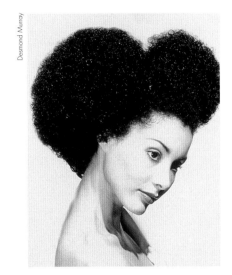

Desmond Murray

The first edition of *African-Caribbean Hairdressing* went a long way towards meeting the needs of lecturers, stylists and students of hairdressing as a reference book covering all aspects of African-Caribbean hair. Since 1998 the industry has continued to grow in strength and I am delighted to introduce the second edition of *African-Caribbean Hairdressing*. The original text has been updated and new step by step photos added for some techniques. The most significant change is the addition of two chapters covering Hair Extensions and Natural Hair. Both are packed full of the latest techniques and step by step illustrations. The techniques are both creative and innovative. All credit goes to Patricia Livingston for her contribution to the development of these two new chapters.

I never cease to be amazed and overwhelmed at the dedication, commitment and talent within the industry without which this book most certainly would not have been possible. Yet again individuals have shown their support in agreeing to share their skills, knowledge and artistry. I cannot thank them enough for their time, enthusiasm and support, each one of them needs special mention: Desmond Murray, Burnet Forbes Salon, Beauty of the Nile, Curlise Dixon, Claudette Thornton, Hibiscus Hair Salon, Vinetta Mcintosh and Shantae's Hair Salon.

Finally, I hope you find this new edition inspiring, informative and motivating.

Sandra Gittens

Please note: The term African-Caribbean, used throughout this book, refers to people of colour from the black African diaspora in Britain, America, Canada, Europe and Australasia.

Client care

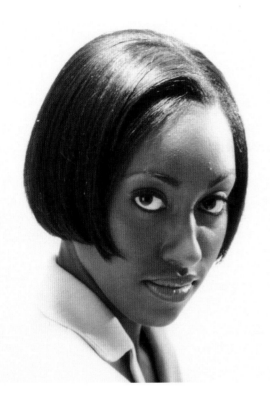

Michell McIntosh for Luster

1

Learning objectives

This chapter covers the following:

- **consultation**
- **analysis**
- **client care**
- **retailing of products**

Consultation

The consultation and analysis process is a *vital* part of any hairdressing service and must be carried out prior to any chemical or hair-care treatment.

Failure to carry out a thorough consultation and analysis could result in the following:

- hair loss and damage to the scalp
- hair breakage
- an unsatisfactory end result.

Incorrect consultation and analysis will most certainly result in a dissatisfied client. Carrying out a thorough consultation and analysis will help you produce a detailed client history, decide on a course of action and identify any previous problems such as:

- clients' requirements and concerns
- scalp irritation
- hair breakage
- past problems with particular products.

The results can be used to develop a programme of hair care treatment for the client. The consultation and analysis

Tip

A record card is filled out to provide detailed information on services carried out. Information recorded on the record card can be used as a reference in the event of:

- providing a client history for the stylist/salon
- scalp irritation and hair breakage
- a dissatisfied client.

Client consultation

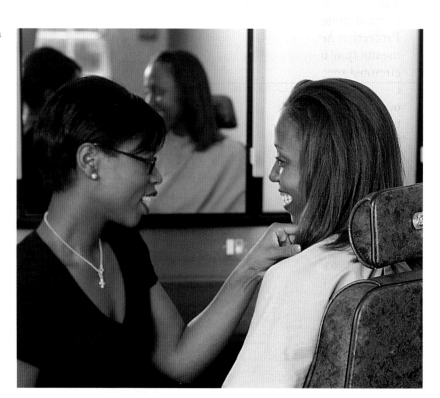

A client record card

CLIENT RECORD CARD

Name:		Address:		

Telephone numbers:	Date first registered:	Age group:	
Home:		☐ 5–15	☐ 16–30
Work:	Stylist:	☐ 31–50	☐ 50+

Hair condition:		Scalp condition:	

Date	Services used	Remarks	Stylist

Tip

Any client information held on consultation sheets or record cards is covered under the Data Protection Act. This means that under no circumstances should clients' details be taken out of the salon or given to another person.

Tip

Always treat each client as an individual. This will give her a feeling of well-being and reassure her that you will take the best possible care with her hair.

process is discussed in depth throughout each technical chapter; see pages 98, 120, 183 and 285 for examples of consultation sheets.

On completion of all hairdressing services a record card should be filled in for each client. The information on the record card must list every technical service, product used, problems experienced and whether or not the client was satisfied with the end result. There should be one record card per client which should be filled in on each visit to the salon.

Above is an example of a typical record card. (For further information on consultation and analysis, see the chapter relating to the chemical process you intend to carry out.)

Creating the correct environment is important when carrying out a consultation or analysis. A quiet area of the salon which has been set aside for the consultation process would be ideal. If this is not possible, make sure the client is sitting in a comfortable chair.

The following points are guidelines to observe when conducting a consultation.

- Eye contact is important: sit on the same level as the client rather than talking to her through the mirror. This will help make the client feel comfortable and relaxed.

- Speak to the client in soft tones to avoid other clients hearing personal information.
- Ask positive questions to elicit the correct information such as:

  'When was your last perm?'

  'Was your scalp sensitive at any time during the process?'

  'Was there any breakage?'
- Do not ask closed questions such as:

  'So your last perm was okay?' as this may provoke the response 'Yes' and not highlight any problems that might have occurred during and after the process.

Analysis

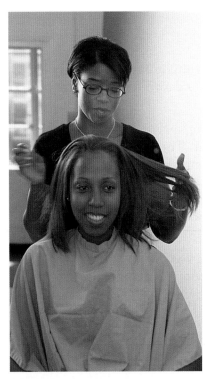

Analysis

Once you have completed the consultation, begin the analysis of the scalp and hair. Comb the hair from the ends, working up the mid-lengths to the roots. Start at the back of the head and work up to the front hairline.

This will allow you to observe and make an assessment of the following areas:

- the condition of the scalp and hair
- whether there is hair loss or breakage
- hair texture
- density
- elasticity
- porosity.

As part of your analysis you should carry out the following tests, especially when the hair is going to be chemically processed:

Hair texture

This identifies how thick or thin the hair is. Hair texture falls into three categories:

- thick/coarse
- medium/normal
- fine/thin.

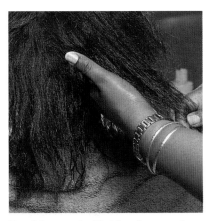

Looking at individual strands of hair

Test to determine hair texture

Select a few strands of hair and hold between the fingers. Look at each individual strand of hair and decide how thick or thin the hair is (see illustration).

Density

Density is the number of hairs per square inch of the head. For example, you might have fine hair but if you have a lot of it, the density will be thick even though the individual hairs are fine.

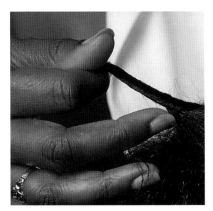

Twisting the hair to determine density

Test to determine hair density

Section approximately one square inch of hair on the scalp and twist the hair. This will give you an indication of how dense the hair is, e.g. thick, medium or thin (see illustration).

Elasticity

This is the ability of the hair to stretch and return to its own length without breaking.

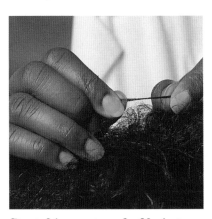

Stretching a strand of hair to determine elasticity

Test to determine elasticity

Select a strand of hair and hold it between the index finger and thumb of one hand at least 12.5 mm (0.5 inches) away from the scalp. With the index finger and thumb of the other hand hold the hair near mid-length, leaving no more than 40 mm (1.5 inches) of hair between each finger. Stretching the hair between each finger and thumb will give an indication of the amount of stretch/elasticity the hair has. It will also indicate how strong or weak the hair is. If the hair snaps while stretching it has poor elasticity and is weak. If it stretches and goes back to its own length it has good elasticity and is strong (see illustration).

Porosity

This is the ability of the hair to take in moisture.

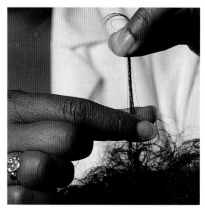

Sliding the fingers along the hair to determine porosity

Tip

A combination of looking at and feeling the hair will help you come to a decision on the condition. For example, if the hair has a dry, discoloured appearance along with feeling dry this is usually an indication of over-processed, damaged hair.

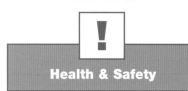

Health & Safety

Never carry out any hairdressing process if you think there is an infestation or infection present which could be contagious. It is important that you do not put other clients at risk. Always get a second opinion if you are unsure. Having confirmed the presence of an infection or infestation, advise your client to seek medical advice. Be tactful in your approach; take your client aside and inform her out of earshot of other clients.

Test to determine porosity

Hold a few strands of hair between the index finger and thumb at the points. Use the index finger and thumb of the other hand to slide up and down the strands of hair. The rougher or bumpier the surface or cuticle of the hair feels, the more damaged or porous the hair is. Hair in good condition has a smooth feel (see illustration).

(For further information on hair tests see Chapter 2 and the technical chapter that relates to the chemical process you are intending to carry out.)

Checking for infestations and infections

During your analysis you should ensure there are no infestations, infections or non-infectious conditions present.

Infestations

- head lice
- scabies.

Infections

- ringworm
- impetigo.

Non-infectious conditions

- traction alopecia
- alopecia
- dandruff
- psoriasis.

(For further information on infestations, infections and non-infectious conditions found on the skin and scalp, see Chapter 15.)

On completion of the analysis you will be able to make a diagnosis of your client's scalp, hair texture and hair condition. The result of your analysis will help you decide:

- whether the scalp and hair are healthy, and whether the hair is strong enough to be chemically processed
- the strength of product to be used
- the type of product to be selected
- the method or technique to be used.

Client care

As a stylist it is important to develop a professional approach when dealing with clients. Your client should feel confident that you have the knowledge and experience to take care of her hair. A client who has confidence in the stylist could become a loyal customer. A successful stylist is one who has clients who return time after time. Loyal clients are gained over the years for the following reasons:

- a good professional manner and approach
- excellent hairdressing skills
- product and technical knowledge
- good client care
- a fair policy for dealing with customer complaints.

A professional manner and approach

Presenting yourself in a professional manner is important. Always remember – first impressions count. The way you look or behave can either attract or lose clients. The following points should be observed as a professional hairdresser:

- personal appearance
- personal hygiene
- attitude towards clients and colleagues
- the way you conduct yourself.

Make sure you look the part. Your hair must be clean, well cut and styled. As a hairdresser you can help promote new looks and fashion trends. Your look could inspire the client to change the style or colour of her hair. Your clothes should be clean and fresh every day. It is important to avoid body odour by bathing daily and using deodorant. Teeth should be brushed regularly to avoid bad breath. Hands and nails should be well groomed. Use barrier and hand creams to protect and moisturise your hands.

Conduct is also important. As a professional hairdresser you should:

- always work in a proficient and professional manner
- be respectful and loyal to your clients, colleagues and employer
- never chew, smoke, eat or drink when working on clients' hair

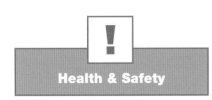

Health & Safety

If you have a cut or abrasion on your hands it is important that you cover it to avoid cross-infection.

- always be pleasant while working in the salon
- avoid being aggressive or argumentative – poor body language can send the wrong messages to clients
- make sure you give the client your undivided attention during her time in the salon
- never carry on conversations or gossip with other colleagues while working on clients' hair
- treat all clients in the same way – do not openly show any favouritism
- always observe health and safety guidelines when working in the salon.

Tip

Reading and subscribing to trade magazines can also be used as a means of keeping abreast with changing trends.

Maintaining good hairdressing skills

As a hairdresser it is important that you maintain and update your skills by attending the following whenever possible:

- technical workshops
- demonstrations
- product company seminars
- lectures.

Stylists that do not keep up to date and informed of changing trends could lose their clients or become bored with doing the same type of work. This could lead to a lack of motivation. As a stylist it is your responsibility to motivate both yourself and the client.

It is also important to create variety and interest in your daily work by introducing your client to:

- a new hairstyle
- a new hair cut
- a change in hair colour
- new products available on the market.

If you are not aware of current fashions and looks you will not be able carry out any of the above.

Good client care

It is important that you create the correct environment for customers. The salon must always be clean and tidy. Make sure you tidy and clean as you work. Do not leave used

Tip

It is good practice at regular intervals throughout the hairdressing process to enquire and check that your client is comfortable.

Always use clean towels and gowns on clients to avoid cross-infection. (For further information see Chapter 15.)

Avoid accidents in the salon by cleaning up any spillage and sweeping up hair cuttings immediately.

towels and gowns around the salon – once used they should be put into laundry bins and laundered immediately.

How we welcome the client is of great importance. Following the guidelines listed below will assist you in providing quality client care.

- Attend to the client immediately on their arrival at the salon.
- Always greet the client with a smile.
- Help the client to remove outer garments such as a jacket or a coat.
- Assist the client to put on a gown and other outer protection.
- Offer the client refreshment such as coffee, tea, water or a cold drink.

Tip

Always refer to the client by name. This will make her feel you have a special interest in her. Use the first or last name depending on how well you know the client or according to the salon policy. Do not refer to the client as 'she' or ' he' as this can come across as being extremely rude.

A knowledge of services on offer

It is important that you are aware of every service that the salon offers. For example, the price of each treatment, what it entails and the approximate time it will take. Be aware of any promotional offers the salon may be launching so that clients can be kept informed.

Dealing with customer complaints

Always be polite and listen to any complaints or concerns clients may have. These can be:

- prior to any process being given
- during the process
- after any process is carried out.

A good salon will be one which has a policy for dealing with customer complaints and resolving them to the satisfaction

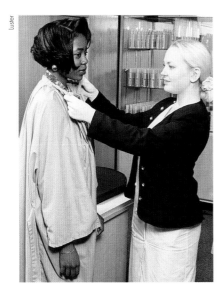

Stylist gowning the client

Tip

Be honest with the client if, after any process, the results are not what you expected. Tell her immediately and offer to carry out corrective treatment. Remember, a breakdown in communication between stylist and client can result in problems and misunderstanding regarding the service, e.g. colour, cut, relaxer, hairstyle achieved.

of the client. Salons with no such policy will eventually lose clients through dissatisfaction. Clients are the reason we exist as hair stylists. A busy salon is one where loyal clients return time after time to the same stylist.

Client complaints can be kept to a minimum by ensuring the following procedures are always carried out:

- Make a thorough consultation and analysis.
- Determine the client's exact requirements prior to commencing any service.
- Confirm the look, technique, chemical treatment and style that the client requires.
- Check with the client that they are comfortable with the colour, cut, perm, etc. both during and after the process.
- Make sure that there is an efficient client booking system to avoid double booking.
- Do not take complaints personally or in a negative way.

The guidelines listed above have been mentioned throughout this chapter and will establish good practice while working in the salon. A dissatisfied client who has had her complaint dealt with effectively by the salon can become one of your most loyal customers.

Clients' complaints and concerns should be dealt with in a positive manner. A typical procedure for dealing with customer complaints is as follows. If a client wishes to make a complaint:

Tip

By dealing immediately with concerns or complaints you are reassuring the client that you care. Never allow a dissatisfied client to leave the salon without resolving the problem.

- take her to a quiet area of the salon
- listen carefully to her concerns or complaint
- take immediate action by correcting any faults or mistakes where possible
- do not become aggressive or rude to her while dealing with the complaint
- do not allow her concerns or complaints to go unnoticed.

Retailing

When clients come into the salon, it is important that full advantage is taken of the time spent with them. This time should be used to educate the clients on how to care for and maintain their hair. By recommending hair products to the

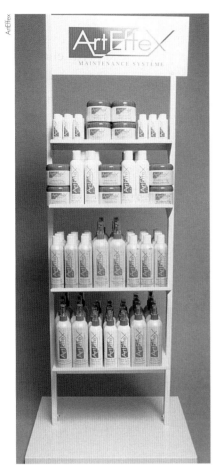

A range of styling products

Tip

Do not put pressure on clients to purchase your products. Although a client may not wish to purchase products immediately, she may buy them at a later date.

client, you are ensuring the hairstyle will be maintained in the best condition.

The following are examples of suitable topics for advice and discussion with your client:

- Discuss the type of products she uses to maintain her hair at home.
- Give advice on how often she should chemically process her hair, for example perming, relaxing, tinting, highlights/lowlights.
- Give advice on how often she should visit the salon for conditioning treatments.
- Discuss how she should maintain her hairstyle between salon visits.
- Recommend a suitable shampoo, conditioner and finishing product that she can use between salon visits. Ideally these should be the same products that you have used on her hair in the salon. Make sure that the cost of the products is made clear to her.

Do not criticise products already used by your client. Always explain in depth why you have recommended a particular product and how the hair will benefit from its use. Advise them to purchase the recommended products once they have used their existing supply but remember that the final decision of whether or not to purchase products rests with the client.

As a stylist, it is important that you keep your clients informed on how to care for their hair. (For further information see Chapters 3 and 6.)

Hair characteristics

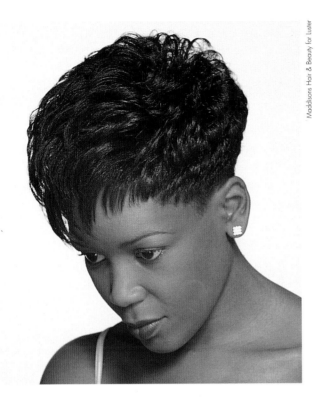

Maddisons Hair & Beauty for Luster

2

Learning objectives

This chapter covers the following:

- hair type
- hair shape
- the structure of the skin
- hair structure
- hair characteristics
- the formation of hair
- chemical properties of the hair
- hair growth
- factors affecting hair growth and development
- diagnostic tests
- effect of water on hair

Hair type

Hairs are thin fibres which cover the majority of the skin surface with the exception of the palms of the hands, the soles of the feet, the lips, the eyelids and the area of skin between the fingers and toes. For differences between the skin of the palms and soles, refer to Chapter 14.

The main function of hair is to act as:

- a buffer to diffuse effects of blows and knocks
- an insulating layer around skin when temperature drops
- a warning mechanism – an indicator to any foreign objects on skin, in ears or nose
- a sense organ – sensitive to touch due to nerve supply connected to each hair follicle
- protection for delicate organs. In these areas, hair is more dense, for example around reproductive organs, brain and underarms.

Tip

Natural hair needs regular moisturising and conditioning treatments. Refer to Chapters 3 and 13 for more information.

Types of hair

Lanugo: Fine downy hair covering the foetus. This is usually lost around the 32nd week of pregnancy. Some babies are born covered with a lot of lanugo hair, but this is lost within the first few weeks.

Vellus hair: Fine, soft hair which replaces lost lanugo hair over most of the infant body, and remains throughout life. Its growth rate is excessively slow. This type of hair can be seen clearly on the faces of some women.

Terminal hair: Coarse hair which covers the scalp, eyebrows, eyelashes, in ears and nose, under arms, legs, pubic areas and, in men, the chest and face.

Hair which has not been subjected to chemical processes is referred to as **Virgin hair**.

straight hair	wavy hair	curly hair
round	flat, oval	kidney

Cross-section of hair

Ethnic hair groups

- **Caucasian** – loosely waved or straight hair
- **African-Caribbean** – tight curly, or wavy hair
- **Asian** – normal coarse, straight hair.

Hair Shape

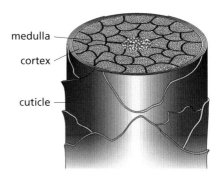

medulla
cortex
cuticle

The hair shaft

The hair shaft varies in shape. Hair shape in cross-section varies according to the curl type, i.e. straight, wavy or curly. Asian hair is typically circular in cross-section. In European hair the shape varies from oval to kidney while Afro hair tends to have more of a flat, oval shape.

The hair above and below the surface of the skin is known as the **hair shaft**. It is divided into three layers: **cuticle**, **cortex** and **medulla**.

Hair is seen in most cultures as our crowning glory and an adornment. How our hair looks can influence how we feel and our self image, hence the term 'bad hair day'. This relatively recent expression reflects the importance which we as individuals attach to how our hair looks and to our ability to style and control hair.

If our hair does not look good this can affect how we portray ourselves to other individuals. A 'bad hair day' could make someone feel unkempt, less confident and not in control. However, this may not be the image that is being portrayed to other people.

As hairstylists, we must have an awareness of the psychological effects that hair and self-image have on the client and their perception of themselves.

If we are going to give the correct advice to clients on hair care treatments it is important that we are knowledgeable about the structure of the skin and hair. An in-depth knowledge of the functions of the skin and hair is necessary if we are going to make a correct diagnosis during consultation and analysis. Knowledge in this area will mean that the correct guidance and recommendations on hair maintenance and the use of aftercare products will be given.

Hair and hair follicles are appendages of the scalp and skin much like nails, sweat glands and sebaceous glands. The hair is fed by a rich supply of blood found in the skin via a network of capillaries. The skin is slightly acid, with a pH between 4.5 and 5.5 which helps protect it against bacteria.

The skin is extremely flexible and covers and protects the whole body. The hair found on the body varies, depending on where it is. Thicker terminal hair is found on the scalp and thinner downy hair found above the lips.

The structure of the skin

The skin is composed of three main layers. The **epidermis** is the top layer of skin that can be seen. It differs in thickness depending on the area of the body that it supports. Epidermal skin is at its thinnest on the eyelids and is thickest on the palms of the hands and the soles of the feet. The central structure of the skin is called the **dermis**. Suspended in the dermis are blood vessels, nerve endings, hair follicles, sweat glands and their ducts, sebaceous glands and papillary muscles. The dermis is composed of collagen, elastin and fibroblast cells. The job of collagen is to support and add bulk to the skin. Elastin is there to give the skin its elasticity which allows the skin to

Structure of the skin

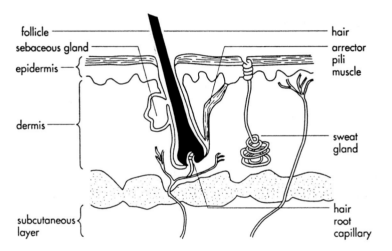

Layers of the epidermis

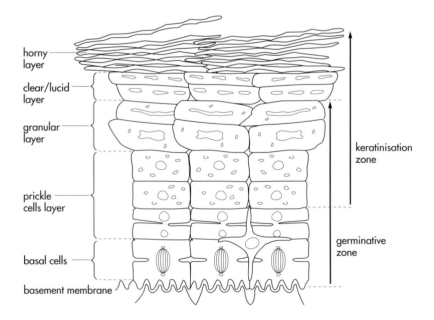

expand and contract like an elastic band. Fibroblast cells manufacture the collagen and elastin fibres.

The third layer of the skin is the **subcutaneous layer** or the fatty layer which helps provide insulation.

The epidermis is made up of five further layers. The most superficial of these five layers is the **horny/cornified** layer followed by the **clear/lucid** layer, the **granular** layer, the **prickle cell** layer and finally the **germinative** layer. Each of these layers has individual characteristics. The table gives an outline of the layers of the epidermis.

Layers of the epidermis

Name	*Description*
Horny (stratum corneum)	Most superficial layers are constantly shed; made up of several layers of keratinised epithelial cells closely packed together; in African-Caribbean skins this layer is thicker and pigment is present; in Caucasian skins no pigment is present in this layer.
Clear/lucid (stratum lucidium)	Small, closely packed transparent cells with no nucleus; this layer is very shallow on the face, and is much thicker on the palms of the hands and the soles of the feet; in Caucasian skin the destruction of melanin is completed here.
Granular (stratum granulosum)	Keratinisation is complete here (living cells containing a nucleus have been changed into flattened layers of cells composed of keratin); the nucleus begins to break down, becoming flatter, and cells are transforming into keratin due to fluid loss.
Prickle cell (stratum spinosum)	Keratinisation begins here.
Germinative (stratum germinativum)	Due to the lower cells being attached to the dermis, fluids are passed from the blood vessels; mitosis, the development of new cells, happens here and gradually the older cells are pushed towards the skin's surface and later shed; melanocytes, melanin-producing cells, are developing here; the concentration of pigment in this layer is significantly greater in African-Caribbean skins as opposed to the concentration in Caucasian skin (for further information on mitosis, see Chapter 2).

Melanin is a brown pigment found in the germinative layer of the epidermis (also found in the horny layer in African-Caribbean skin). When ultraviolet light stimulates the pigmented cells, the brown colour is transmitted to the skin's surface. Melanin acts as the skin's natural protector against the ultraviolet rays of the sun. It helps to filter the **UVA** and **UVB** rays that can be extremely damaging. UVA activates the melanin to produce a short-term, rapid tan and due to its deep penetration, premature ageing is caused. UVB activates vitamin D production and melanin, offering a more long-term tan but is the cause of sunburn which can lead to forms of skin cancer, one of which is **malignant melanoma**.

Hair structure

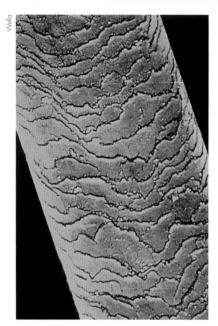

Wella

The hair cuticle

The cuticle

The **cuticle** is the outer layer of the hair. Its main function is to protect the cortex. The cuticle scales are elongated, flattened and overlap each other from the roots to the tips (the same as tiles on a roof). The cuticle makes up 10% of the hair's weight.

The scales are colourless, translucent and easily damaged. A healthy cuticle surface will reflect light, making the hair glossy and shiny. It will feel smooth when felt from roots to ends. An unhealthy cuticle will not reflect light, making the hair look dull. The cuticle scales are raised and feel rough when felt from roots to ends. This is the case with porous or over-processed hair. Curly hair may look dull and feel rough to touch. This is due to the cuticle scales not lying flat, as they follow the crests and waves of the curl contour – some of the cuticle scales will be open. This causes the rays of light to be diffused.

The number of cuticle layers differs between ethnic groups. In Caucasian hair there are normally four to seven layers, Afro seven to eleven layers, Asian eleven or more, thus making this hair type more resistant to chemicals.

The cortex

The **cortex** makes up the main bulk of hair. It contributes to at least three quarters of the hair strength and is home to all the chemical bonds (sulphur bonds, salt bonds and hydrogen bonds) and colour molecules (eumelanin and pheomelanin, for example). The cortical cells are long and thin and composed of small bundles of **macrofibrils**. These are made up of bunches of even smaller **microfibrils**, which in turn are made up of bunches of **protofibrils**, all held together by cross bonds. These bonds determine the elasticity, texture and curl of the hair.

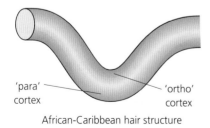

'para' cortex   'ortho' cortex

African-Caribbean hair structure

The cortex of African-Caribbean hair

A cross-section of African-Caribbean hair will show how flat the cortex is, in comparison with Caucasian and Asian hair. The flatter the hair, the faster it will absorb chemicals. The cortical thickness will also vary. This is why African-Caribbean hair is easily damaged.

African-Caribbean hair has both a para and ortho cortex.

- **Para cortex:** the cortical fibres grow in an even, uniformed cylinder; the cells are tightly packed together. Present in straight hair, European and Asian hair. The hair will absorb liquids at an even rate.

- **Ortho cortex:** the cortical fibres grow in an uneven formation following the contours of the wave and curl. Present in curly hair. The hair will absorb liquids at an uneven rate.

Wavy hair has a partly para cortex. The cortex of African-Caribbean curly hair is a combination of para and ortho cortex – the para cortex develops on the outside of the curl and the ortho cortex is present on the inside of the curl. Close examination of a strand of curly hair clearly shows the para and ortho-cortex, in that some sections of a single strand will be thinner than others.

The medulla

The **medulla** is the central core of the hair, consisting of rigid tunnels of cells filled with air spaces running either continuously or intermittently through the hair. A medulla is present in most types of hair, with the exception of very thin hair.

Hair characteristics

In describing the characteristics of hair we refer to type, texture, elasticity, porosity, density and natural curl and shape.

Texture

fine
to medium
fine medium medium to coarse coarse

Hair texture

The **texture** of hair is influenced by the thickness of each individual strand. It is measured by taking the average diameter of a single strand, which is due mainly to its cortex. Texture plays an important part in the choice of chemical applications and the selection of styles.

Resistant hair

Resistant hair has over 12 layers of cuticle, tightly packed together, thus making penetration into the cortex by chemical agents more difficult.

Elasticity

Elasticity is the ability of hair to stretch and return to its natural state without breaking. When dry it will stretch by only 5–10%, when wet it can stretch by up to 60%. Chemical processes such as relaxing, bleaching and permanent waving (curly perms) decrease the elastic properties of hair by up to 25%.

Tensile strength

Tensile strength is the force required to stretch a hair until it breaks. The strength is considerably reduced in hair that is chemically over-processed, for example when previously bleached hair is relaxed. The chemical process decreases the strength to such an extent that the hair becomes very weak and easily broken. In particular, wet hair that has been chemically treated can be very fragile and must be handled with extreme care.

Tip

Always test re-growth area separately.

Porosity

Porosity is the ease or rate at which hair absorbs liquids. Hair in good condition has tightly closed cuticle scales. This presents a hard, smooth surface which protects the cortical fibres, making the absorption of liquids difficult. When the cuticle scales become damaged due to harsh handling and/or chemical abuse, the surface will feel rough where the cuticle scales remain open or are broken, torn or split. The hair will absorb liquids at a much faster rate in these areas, making successful chemical processing impossible, because porous areas of the hair will process faster than non-porous areas.

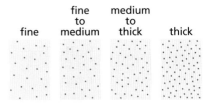

fine   fine to medium   medium to thick   thick

Hair density

Density

Density is a measurement of the number of hairs per square inch of the scalp. On an average adult head there are 100,000–120,000 hair follicles. Hair having a sparse covering is referred to as **thin**; hair having a dense covering is **thick**.

Curl pattern

The **curl pattern** of hair is genetically determined before birth (see Hereditary influences on page 27). The more bent and coiled the hair follicle is, the tighter the curl pattern with the bulb being virtually upside down in very curly hair.

Tip

Part the hair from crown to nape. Place both hands on either side of the parting and release. The rate at which the parting springs close will indicate the tightness of the curl formation.

Hairdressers recognise over 32 different curl patterns, ranging from a very tight spiral curl to a very loose wave. On close examination, there may be three or more varying curl patterns on one head. Areas to note are the hairline, crown, nape, occipital and temple areas. You will find a variety of curl patterns (from wavy to tight curly) throughout the African-Caribbean hair types, whether in Africa, Europe, the Caribbean or North and South America. Hair will also vary in curl pattern due to inter-racial marriage. (You must always carry out a consultation to determine the natural curl pattern prior to processing the hair.)

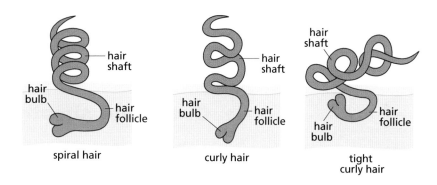

Different curl patterns respond to chemicals in various ways. Establishing the more resistant curl formation is an important factor when selecting suitable relaxer and curl re-arranger strengths. (For more information see Chapters 7 and 8.)

The formation of hair

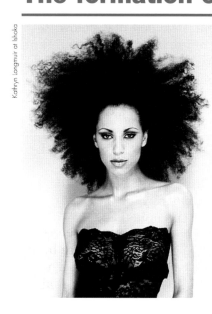

The hair **follicle** grows from an indentation of the epidermis into the dermis. Follicles are normally found in clusters of three. Each follicle is about 4 mm deep and 0.4 mm wide, with the base widening out into a **bulb**. The walls of the follicle are made up of layers of connective tissue. Each follicle has its own sebaceous gland that opens into the follicle, lubricating the hair inside. Beneath the sebaceous gland is the **arrector pili** muscle that is connected to the nerve fibres.

The follicle wall has three layers:

- **inner root sheath** – which is actually part of the growing hair
- **outer root sheath**
- **connective tissue sheath**.

Inner root sheath

The **inner root sheath** consist of three layers:

- the **henles layer** which is one cell thick
- the **huxleys layer** which is two or more cells thick
- the **cuticle layer** which is made of scales which point downwards and interlock with the cuticle scales of the hair itself which points upwards. It is this interlocking which holds the hair in the hair follicle.

The inner root sheath grows from the **germinative layer**. It disintegrates halfway up the hair follicle around the sebaceous gland opening, leaving the hair to travel up to the epidermis.

Outer root sheath

The **outer root sheath** forms the structural foundation of the hair follicle walls, surrounding and protecting the inner root sheath. The thickness will depend on the diameter of the hair follicle. Above the upper bulb, the outer root sheath is composed of three layers and is at its thickest one third of the way up the length of the hair follicle. Its structure closely resembles that of the epidermis, of which it is actually a part. The **vitreous membrane** separates connective tissue from the outer root sheath.

Connective tissue sheath

The **connective tissue sheath** provides a constant blood supply to nourish the hair follicle. Attached just below the sebaceous gland is a network of nerve endings, surrounding and penetrating the connective tissue. These detect different types of stimuli, for example temperature, pain and pressure.

Arrector pili muscle

The **arrector pili muscle** is a long tissue that extends from the outer root sheath about one third of the way up the hair follicle to the underside of the epidermis. In cold temperatures or when we experience fear, the muscle contracts and pulls the sloping hair follicle into an erect position. The erect hair traps a warm layer of air above the skin. The skin near to the follicle opening becomes raised, causing a 'goose bump' appearance. The muscle also acts as a warning device to detect the presence of small insects crawling on the skin.

Sweat glands

Sweat glands or **sudoriferous glands** cover the entire skin surface. Sweat is a watery secretion, 98% water and 2% salt. Perspiration occurs due to the discharge of the solution into long, slim ducts and then onto the skin through tiny openings called pores. The sweat cools the skin by evaporation.

There are two types of sweat glands. The smaller glands are called **eccrine** glands. They are independent of the hair follicle and open directly on to the skin surface. They produce a watery secretion, which can be controlled by regular washing and daily use of deodorants.

The larger glands are known as **apocrine** glands. These glands are attached to the follicle wall and open into the mouth of the follicle. They produce a waxy, milky emulsion, responsible for body odour. The odour can be controlled by regular washing and daily use of anti-perspirant.

Sebaceous glands

Sebaceous glands are often referred to as oil glands. They are attached to the hair follicle and produce an anti-bacterial, waxy oil called **sebum** directly into the hair follicle, coating the surface of hair and skin.

A thin layer of sebum adds lustre and sheen to hair and skin. When the production of sebum is excessive the hair becomes lank and greasy, often seen in the nape area of wavy hair. However, under-production of sebum causes hair and skin to look and feel very dry and dull. This is more common in tight-curly hair, as sebum cannot successfully coat the hair when there are sharp bends and twists in the curl pattern. The curlier the hair, the longer it takes for sebum to travel up the hair shaft and lubricate the hair.

Hair colour

Natural hair colour is genetically predetermined before birth, but it can be lightened or darkened artificially by chemical treatments. Cells called **melanocytes**, which develop in the germinal matrix, produce granules of colour molecules called **melanin**. These colour molecules are evenly distributed throughout the cortex.

The colour largely depends on the amount of pigment production by the melanocytes. Pigments form the natural colour tones of the hair. They are usually **yellow**, **brown**, **red**, **indigo** or **orange**.

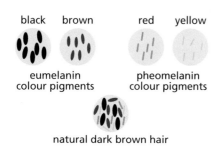

black   brown   red   yellow

eumelanin   pheomelanin
colour pigments   colour pigments

natural dark brown hair

There are two main types of melanin:

- **Eumelanin:** oval shaped black and brown granules found in large quantities in dark hair.
- **Pheomelanin:** long, thin, red and yellow granules found in small quantities throughout the cortex of fair hair.

Albinism

Failure of melanocytes to produce colour pigments in hair and skin results in a congenital condition called **albinism**. An albino has creamy white skin colour, yellowish-white to yellowish-red hair colour and pink eyes. (For further information see Chapter 11.)

Grey hair

Grey hair is a mixture of coloured and white hair. This condition is normally a result of the ageing process, but can also occur as a result of medication and illness, leading to the absence of melanocytes in rejuvenated hair follicles, producing colourless hairs.

Chemical properties of hair

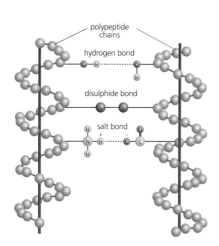

polypeptide chains

hydrogen bond

disulphide bond

salt bond

Polypeptide chains, showing linking bonds

Hair, nails and the horny outer layer of the epidermis are all made up of a protein called **keratin**. Smaller units called **amino acids** combine in various formulas, creating different types of protein. About **22** amino acids form proteins. They consist of atoms of the following elements in these proportions:

- carbon 50%
- oxygen 21%
- nitrogen 18%
- hydrogen 7%
- sulphur 4%

Amino acids are joined together by **peptide bonds** to produce long **polypeptide chains**, which coil and fold like springs to form a spiral or alpha helix (α helix). In the hair, these spirals lie parallel to each other.

Disulphide/sulphur and cystine bonds are the strongest bonds which form the 'rungs' in a ladder-like structure, holding two polypeptide chains together. These are broken down by chemical relaxers and permanent wave (curly perms). (See Chapters 7 and 8.)

Salt bonds are easily broken by weak acid or alkaline solutions. They are made up of two amino acids with opposite electrical charges. Hydrogen bonds are responsible for the elastic properties of hair. These break when the hair is wet or warmed and reform when it is dried or cools (see Chapters 4 and 5).

Hair growth

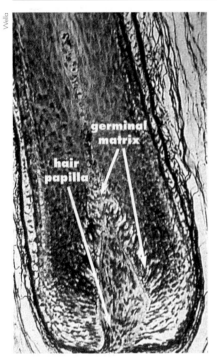

The hair papilla and germinal matrix

Terminal hair has three cycles: **anagen**, **catagen** and **telogen**.

Anagen

Anagen is the growing stage. It can last from 2 to 7 years as the duration of anagen for each hair follicle is genetically predetermined. Hair grows approximately 1.25 cm per month. On an average adult head, 85% of follicles are in anagen at any one time.

The hair grows from the **hair bulb**, which contains the **germinal matrix**. The **dermal papilla** is the capillary network that provides the hair follicle with nourishment.

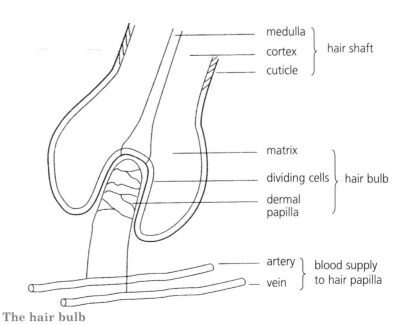

The hair bulb

Germinal matrix

Rapid cell division takes place in the **germinal matrix**. The new cells die and push the old cells upwards. At this stage the newly formed cells arrange themselves into their designated layers, three layers of the hair and three layers of the inner root sheath. One third of the way up the hair follicle they harden, die and become fully **keratinised**, forming keratin.

Catagen

This is the end of the growing period. All activity in the germinal matrix ceases. The blood supply from the dermal papilla is cut off. The lower part of the hair detaches from the base of the follicle, forming a club-ended hair. The hair travels slowly up the hair follicle. The hair follicle shortens to about 1/3 of its natural length. This stage normally lasts for a fortnight. At any one time 1% of follicles are in the catagen stage.

The growth cycle

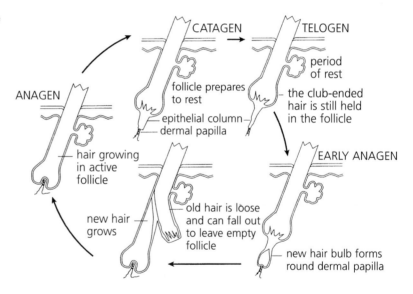

Telogen

This is known as the resting stage, normally lasting 3 to 4 months. There is no activity in the hair follicle. When this period has ended the follicle lengthens. The dermal papilla will provide nourishment, whilst new hair cells start dividing in the germinal matrix. The new growing hair eventually loosens and pushes the old hair out of the follicle. On average, 60–100 hairs are lost daily.

One hair follicle may contain two or more growing hairs. One will be more dominant and larger than the other(s).

Factors affecting hair growth and development

The development of hair can be affected by any of the following factors:

Diet

Our bodies depend on a balanced diet rich in vitamins A, B, C and proteins in order to produce healthy hair and nail growth. The hair shaft itself is dead. The actual nourishment from the dermal papilla goes directly to the newly forming hair cells in the germinal matrix.

Hereditary influences

The characteristics of hair largely depend on the genes passed on from our parents. An offspring receives 23 chromosomes from each parent. These chromosomes influence hair colour, length, texture, natural curl and baldness.

Age

Several changes take place in the hair follicles during our lifetime. At puberty the hair begins to thin, due to the onset of hormone production. Between the ages of 15 and 25, hair growth is at its most rapid, gradually slowing down as we become older. As new hairs replace old ones, they may differ in colour, texture, curl, and thickness. For example, the onset of greying hair.

Climate

In warmer climates, where there is a greater amount of ultraviolet light (sunlight), growth will be accelerated. High, intense ultraviolet light will bleach and dry colour-treated hair (see Chapter 11).

Health

Stress plays an important part in everyday existence. We cannot live without it. Stress reveals itself in many forms: illness, hair loss (alopecia), hair shaft disorders (e.g. monilethrix), headaches, tiredness, exhaustion, digestive problems and panic attacks. It is important to find ways of reducing the levels of stress we encounter. Diet, regular exercise, sleep and relaxation are all factors which influence general health.

Hormones

Hormones influence hair growth and sexual development. The levels of hormones change at different stages in life: during pregnancy, puberty and menopause, all of which can cause diffuse hair fall. There are seven glands in the body that secrete one or more hormones into the blood. Each hormone has a specific function: see the table below.

Effects of disease or illness

Illness and diseases influence the hair growth cycle, by either slowing down or speeding up the growth rate. Such changes can cause hair and colour loss, and general thinning of the hair, which may occur a few months after the illness has passed. A microscopic examination of the hair shaft will reveal evidence of varying degrees of ill health.

Hormonal control and effects on hair

Gland	Hormone	Controls	Effects on hair
Pituitary	Growth hormone; hormones controlling other glands	Regulates growth; increases activity of the glands	Over-production – rapid growth and thickening; under-production – hair loss.
Thyroid	Thyroxine	Influences mental and physical development	Over-production – thinning hair; under-production – dry, coarse, brittle hair in crown area.
Parathyroid	Parathyroid hormone	Regulates calcium levels in the blood	Under-production – causes inferior keratin production causing abnormalities in skin, hair and nails.
Adrenals	Cortex: cortisone medulla: adrenaline	Adrenaline prepares the body for action in an emergency; cortisone regulates the body's use of food	Over-production of cortisone – facial hair in women.
Pancreas	Insulin	Regulates the blood sugar level	
Sex glands			
Ovaries (women)	Oestrogen	Influences secondary sexual characteristics and stimulates ovaries to release egg cells at the onset of puberty	Regulates hair growth at the onset of puberty; increases sebaceous gland activity.
Testes (men)	Testosterone	Stimulates testes to produce sperm at the onset of puberty	Regulates hair growth at the onset of puberty; increases sebaceous gland activity.

Medication

Some drugs used to control an illness can cause hair loss or baldness, for example the extreme hair loss which results from chemotherapy cancer treatment.

Pregnancy

During pregnancy, many of the hair follicles which are due to enter catagen continue in anagen, therefore naturally increasing the density of the hair. When the levels of hormones fall after birth, these hair follicles all enter catagen at the same time, causing an excessive and potentially alarming hair fall.

Substance abuse

The continuous abuse of drugs and alcohol can cause premature hair loss. The body becomes abused, and vital organs and the body systems function erratically. In extreme cases, these organs will eventually shut down.

Diagnostic tests

Diagnostic tests are performed in order to support and confirm previously established diagnosis. Not all tests are required for all clients. However, elasticity and porosity tests can be classified as the two basic tests and should always be performed. (For details of these tests see Chapter 1.)

Test curl

A test carried out during permanent waving to check the development of the curl during the process.

Curl test/pre-perm test

A test carried out before a permanent wave to determine the correct strength re-arranger, the roller size and development time.

Incompatibility test

This test is used to determine if there are any metallic salts present on the hair, which might affect a subsequent

Tip

Carry out an incompatibility test on clients who have colour-treated hair with a green or brown hue.

colouring, bleaching or perming process. These salts are contained in colour restorers and enhancers. They react violently with hydrogen peroxide.

Strand test

A test to check the colour development during colouring, bleaching or colour removal.

Test cutting

A test that can be used for colouring, bleaching or relaxing, to determine compatibility.

Skin test/patch test/pre-disposition test

A test to measure the skin's reaction to permanent colouring agents.

The effect of water on hair

Curly hair is generally fragile – when wet it stretches more and is at its weakest. Water lubricates the hair and allows it to be moulded and shaped. Hair is **hygroscropic**, i.e. it has the ability to absorb and retain moisture.

In a dry atmosphere, the hair loses moisture and becomes dry. In humid conditions the hair absorbs moisture and becomes lank. For example, when virgin hair is hot-combed, curled or set it will last longer in a dry atmosphere.

Healthy hair retains 15% of water, trapped in small spaces within the cortical fibres. Water molecules adhere to the hydrogen bonds and increase the elasticity. As the hair absorbs moisture it swells. The degree of expansion depends largely on damage to the cortical fibres. If there is excessive damage to cuticle and cortex, the hair will become more porous and swell a great deal more compared to that of healthy cuticle and cortex. As a result of this it will take longer to dry.

Shampooing and conditioning

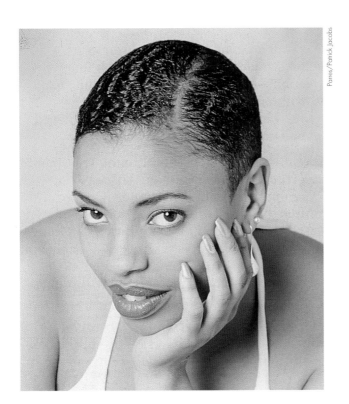

Parres/Patrick Jacobs

3

Learning objectives

This chapter covers the following:

- **the purpose of shampooing hair**

- **shampooing technique**

- **conditioners and conditioning treatments**

- **massage techniques**

One of the most important services carried out in a salon is **shampooing**. Cleansing the hair is the starting point from which most of the services we provide in the salon begin – a head of hair not properly cleansed during the shampooing process could spell disaster for any following service(s). A client who is aware that her hair has not been properly cleansed will be unhappy and discontented throughout her time in the salon.

Shampooing is the start of good customer care. A good shampoo will set the standard of hair care which follows. Hair that is not shampooed properly will be difficult to style, brittle, and will have an odour. Once the hair is cleansed thoroughly, the maximum result will be achieved with all following hairdressing processes.

The use of conditioners and regular conditioning treatments are extremely important when working on African-Caribbean hair. The application of conditioner is important regardless of whether the hair is in its natural state or chemically processed. It is important to condition the hair after each shampoo or chemical process. African-Caribbean hair lacks moisture and needs to be conditioned on a regular basis. Regular conditioning treatments will replace moisture lost during chemical and styling processes.

Using the correct conditioner on African-Caribbean hair will make the hair more manageable and reduce breakage. The benefits of conditioning treatments will be discussed in depth in this chapter.

The purpose of shampooing hair

We shampoo hair to:

- remove sebum, grime, dirt, dead skin and sweat
- remove product build-up
- stimulate the scalp
- relax the client prior to other processes.

Tip

Over-shampooing can cause harm by drying out the scalp and hair. This could lead to a dry scalp condition.

Some of the products used on African-Caribbean hair leave a build-up on the hair which attracts particles of dust, dirt and general pollution found in the atmosphere. It is important that the hair is shampooed thoroughly to remove all debris and product build-up.

A good shampoo should cleanse the scalp and hair without stripping out all the natural oils and moisture. The hair should also be left relatively tangle-free in preparation for the conditioner.

Shampoos are of two types:

- **soap**
- **soap-free**.

Soap-based shampoos are no longer used in hairdressing. They are alkaline and in hard water they form a scum and leave a build-up on the hair. The hair will look dull, dry and feel coarse to the touch. Applying a chemical to hair that has been treated with a soap-based shampoo will result in hair breakage.

A rinse made with **citric acid** (lemon juice) or **acetic acid** (vinegar) in water will remove build-up caused by using a soap-based shampoo. Alternatively use a product which will remove any alkaline deposits left on the hair. The hair will regain its shine and look healthy.

As part of the treatment the hair should be shampooed with a soap-free shampoo. These are usually slightly acidic, and cleanse as well as helping to remove any alkaline build-up.

Surface tension

To be able to cleanse the hair effectively, a shampoo has to act as a wetting agent. Water on its own is no good at wetting the hair. It tends to form globules on the surface of the hair or just run off. This is due to **surface tension**. To allow the hair to become wet, the surface tension has to be broken. This is done when the shampoo is added to the water.

Cleansing action of shampoo

The detergents used in shampoo are made up of special, rather long molecules. One end of the molecule is attracted to grease: it is **hydrophobic**. The other is attracted to water: it is **hydrophilic**.

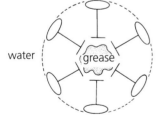

Detergent molecules surrounding grease

A detergent molecule

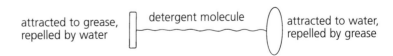

When water with detergent is put on a greasy surface such as hair, the end of the molecule which repels water attaches itself to the grease and removes it from the surface. This loosens any debris, which is also removed by the shampooing action. The grease and loosened debris can then be rinsed away.

Tip

The pH scale is used to measure acidity and alkalinity. 7 on the pH scale is neutral. Anything below 7 is acid and anything above 7 is alkaline.

Tip

Over use of a shampoo/ conditioner is wasteful – excess product is washed down the shampoo basin. Only use the manufacturer's recommended amount.

Tip

It is rare to find an oily condition in African-Caribbean hair (see Chapter 2 for further information). If you do come across a head of hair with this problem, or that has a build-up of products that are not easily removed by a normal shampoo, use a shampoo that will remove the oil first, followed by a moisturising shampoo to avoid over-drying the hair.

Types of shampoos

Most shampoos used on African-Caribbean hair have a neutral pH of 7 or just below. pH-balanced shampoo will have a kinder effect on the hair, leaving it tangle-free and in good condition. The softer the water, the better the final result. The shampoo easily will form a lather which will retain the foam for a few seconds.

In hard water conditions the shampoo will not lather well nor retain a foam (although we realise today that a shampoo does not need to foam excessively to function properly). A good quality shampoo will require smaller quantities to cleanse the scalp and hair effectively.

Active ingredients used in soap-free shampoos are **triethanolamine lauryl sulphate** and **sodium lauryl sulphate**. These act as a detergent. Shampoo can contain a variety of additives to correct various conditions of the scalp and hair. Some additives contained in treatment shampoos are outlined in the table opposite.

Mineral deposits

Mineral deposits are found in hard water conditions. Rinsing the hair with hard water will leave deposits on the hair after it is dried. These can affect the hair and interfere with further chemical processes. The hair is left dull, lifeless and brittle. There are special shampoos on the market which can be used to cleanse the hair effectively of all deposits.

Consultation and analysis

Before shampooing any head of hair it is important to carry out a thorough client consultation and analysis. This will give you an indication of the type of shampoo to use and any scalp or hair problems that need correcting.

It is important to discuss in depth with your client, any concerns she might have regarding her scalp and hair. Problems that would require a treatment shampoo are:

- dry scalp and hair
- damaged, dry, brittle hair
- dandruff affected scalp
- mineral deposits on hair.

Shampoo	Active ingredients	When to use	When not to use	Problems that can arise
Neutralising	Ammonium lauryl sulphate/citric acid – conditioner	After every relaxer	Permed hair	Could cause curl to drop due to acidity.
Dry, damaged hair	Coconut, jojoba, almond or mineral oils, hydrolysed protein, amino acid	On damaged, dry breaking hair or as a pre-treatment shampoo. Natural hair	Before a perm	Could cause a barrier and prevent penetration of perm lotion.
De-tangling/ conditioning, combined shampoo and conditioning	Cationic based shampoo acts as a detergent and conditioner	Extremely porous, damaged hair as a pre-treatment shampoo. Natural hair	Prior to a perm	Difficult to rinse out; clings to the hair; can cause a build-up and form a barrier to other services; will not cleanse the hair sufficiently and is not effective as a conditioner; will still need to use additional conditioner after shampooing.
Moisturising (a good moisturising shampoo will not form a build-up)	Hydrolised protein, amino acid, oil such as: coconut, jojoba, almond, mineral	Dry, damaged hair prior to applying conditioning treatment as a de-tangler. Natural hair		
Dandruff (pityriasis capitis)	Zinc pyrithione	Dandruff infected scalp	Prior to a perm or relaxer	On African Caribbean hair can have an extremely drying effect on the scalp and hair; alternate with a normal conditioning shampoo; do not use before perming or relaxing as this could cause scalp irritation.
	Selenium sulphide	As above. Prescribed by a doctor – only use on severe cases of dandruff	As above	Prolonged use can cause dermatitis; can make African-Caribbean hair dry and brittle.

Consultation

1 Prepare the client for consultation by putting on a gown and towels.

2 De-tangle the hair using a large tooth comb.

3   Make a thorough assessment of the hair as you comb through.

4   Discuss any concerns you may have about the hair and scalp with your client.

5   Discuss the type of cleansing, conditioning and aftercare products used.

6   Provide feedback to your client on your analysis and recommend suitable products.

7   Fill in a record card on products used.

Analysis

1   Comb the hair and observe if any hair is coming out from the scalp or breaking during combing.

2   Look at the scalp to ensure it is healthy.

3   Look at the condition of the scalp and hair to ensure it is not dry and there is no build-up of finishing products.

4   Fill in a record card on products used based on the results of your analysis.

Shampooing technique

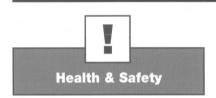

Health & Safety

It is important to make sure that any massage technique is carried out gently but firmly, to avoid any damage.

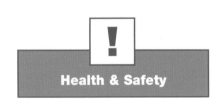

Health & Safety

Make sure the water used to shampoo is not too hot, as this could scald the scalp.

The shampooing process is made effective by the combination of the **shampoo** and **massage** technique. The purpose of massaging the scalp during the shampooing process is to assist the removal of grease, dirt and debris. It is important to make sure the technique used lifts the dirt and cleanses without being abrasive. Massaging the scalp roughly can cause breakage and damage to the scalp and hair.

There are two main massage movements used when shampooing the hair:

● **Effleurage** is a gentle, stroking movement used when applying shampoo or rinsing the hair.

● **Petrissage** is a circular, kneading, lifting movement used when massaging and cleansing the scalp and hair.

Shampooing process

1   Follow steps 1 to 7 in consultation and 1 to 4 in analysis.

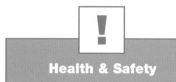

Health & Safety

Make sure the basin is clean before and after use to avoid the risk of cross-infection.

2 Make sure the client's head rests comfortably in the shampoo basin.

3 Test the water temperature on the back of the hand to make sure the water is not too hot. Always check with the client that she is comfortable with the water temperature, which should be tepid to warm.

4 Wet the hair thoroughly (a).

5 Using the selected shampoo, pour the required amount of shampoo into the palm of the hand. Rub your hands together and distribute the shampoo throughout the hair using circular and stroking movements (b), (c) & (d).

6 Gently push your fingers under the hair and using the ball of your fingers, massage the scalp gently using circular movements (e).

7 Continue to massage the scalp gently by using a petrissage movement throughout the head (f).

8 After massaging the scalp for one to two minutes, rinse the hair thoroughly (g).

9 Apply a second portion of shampoo using the same technique as before. Two applications should be enough to cleanse the hair and scalp properly.

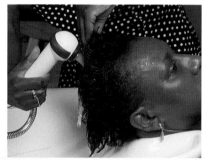

(a) Wetting the hair

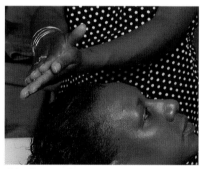

(b) Spreading shampoo over the palms

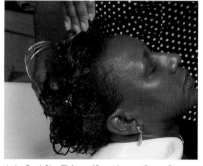

(c) & (d) Distributing the shampoo throughout the hair using effleurage movements

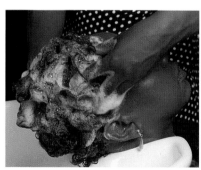

(e) Pushing the fingers under the hair and massaging the scalp

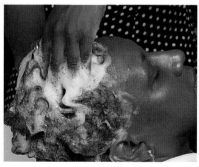

(f) Gently massaging the scalp using a petrissage movement

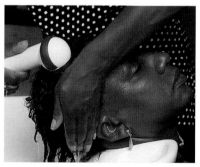

(g) Rinsing the hair

Tip

If the hair is dirty or has product build-up, make a third application. If the hair has been shampooed one or two days before, one application may be sufficient.

Tip

Make sure that the hair is rinsed properly after the final shampoo. Residual shampoo could cause dry, itchy scalp and brittle hair.

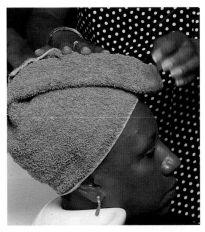

(h) Wrapping a towel around the hair

10 Be careful not to tangle the hair during the shampooing process. This could cause the hair to become damaged and break.

11 Once the hair has been thoroughly cleansed and all the shampoo has been rinsed out, remove the excess water from the hair by wrapping the head with a clean towel (h).

Conditioners and conditioning treatments

Tip

Once hair has been damaged it cannot be repaired. In extreme cases of damage the hair should be cut off. Conditioning treatments will temporarily repair the hair and give it a better feel and appearance, but once shampooed, the hair must be reconditioned. Protein and restructurant treatments can delay the action of breakage, allowing the hair to grow and be cut gradually.

A good conditioner should:

- disentangle the hair and make it soft
- close the cuticle and make the hair smooth
- make the hair appear glossy and bulkier
- control static electricity
- make the hair easy to comb
- moisturise the hair
- strengthen the hair and help to reduce breakage (even if only temporarily)
- be easily rinsed from the hair.

Conditioners fall into three main categories:

- **Surface/external conditioners** work on the cuticle only and make the hair easier to comb. They act as de-tanglers. Surface/external conditioners will not act as a treatment, and have no long-term effect on the hair. These conditioners tend to be used at the backwash, prior to a shampoo and set, wrap set or blow-dry.

Tip

The condition of the hair changes constantly. It is therefore important that on each visit to the salon by your client, a fresh consultation and analysis takes place, so that the correct treatment can be applied.

Health & Safety

Always follow the manufacturer's recommendations on the application, processing and removal of shampoo and conditioning products.

- **Deep-penetrating conditioners** work on the cortex of the hair, conditioning the hair both internally and externally. They will also make the cuticle appear smoother, control breakage, disentangle the hair, add shine and moisture. Also called internal conditioners, these conditioners help to rebuild the cortex of the hair through the addition of protein.

- **Restructurant conditioners** – sometimes called reconstructurants, these conditioners help to temporarily rebuild the disulphide bonds of the hair and so help to control breakage. To do this they contain proteins (amino acids). Restructurants also moisturise the scalp and hair.

Because of the sensitive nature of African-Caribbean hair and strength of the chemicals used to process the hair, conditioning treatments are very important and must be carried out regularly. As a stylist it is your duty to make sure your client's hair is maintained in the best condition.

The following steps must be taken to maintain the condition of the hair:

- Carry out a thorough consultation and analysis.
- Provide feedback to your client as a possible treatment plan.

Conditioner	Active ingredient	When to use	Purpose
Surface conditioner	Citric acid, *oil, quaternary ammonium compound	After a perm, relaxer or permanent colour	Used after a chemical process to close the cuticle; will restore normal pH and act as a de-tangler.
Deep-penetrating conditioner	Hydrolysed protein, *oil	As a treatment on dry, damaged hair, relaxed or permed hair	Adds moisture and sheen to the hair; replaces lost protein; detangles.
Restructurant the conditioner	Quaternary ammonium compound, amino acids, keratin, *oil	On extremely dry, damaged, brittle or over-processed hair	To temporarily rebuild disulphide bonds and reduce breakage by adding amino acids and keratin to the hair; adds moisture and sheen to the hair; ideal after a relaxer or perm; also detangles hair.

*Oil can refer to any one of the following oils: almond oil, coconut oil, jojoba oil, mineral oil, castor oil. Any of these can be used as an additive to shampoo or conditioning treatments.

- Advise your client on how to maintain the condition of her hair

Regularly analyse your client's hair and update your recommendations for treatment as necessary. The table on the previous page is a summary of conditioning treatments and their uses.

Consultation and analysis

Before applying any conditioning treatment, it is important to carry out a consultation and analysis. If you are going to apply a conditioning treatment, make sure that the shampoo used is compatible with the conditioning treatment selected. Consultation and analysis would be best done away from the shampoo basin and in a styling chair. (For further information, see the section on consultation and analysis in Chapter 1.)

As a result of the consultation you should obtain answers to the following questions:

- How often does the client shampoo and condition her hair?
- Does the client visit the salon for professional hair care treatments?
- Has the client had any previous chemical process on her hair?
- Were there any problems that arose after the last chemical process?
- If yes, what were they?
- Is there anything else that the client is concerned about with regard to her hair?

You should now be able to fill out a record card. Combining this information with your analysis will help you come to a decision on which shampoo and conditioning treatment to use.

Analysis

1   Comb the hair starting from the ends, working up through the middle lengths towards the roots.
2   Observe how much hair comes out during combing. This could be an indication of excessive hair being lost from the roots or breakage.
3   Look at the scalp to ensure it is healthy and in good condition.

Tip

Too much protein or over-use of restructurant conditioners can cause the hair to become brittle, dry and to break. It is important that each visit to the salon by the client is treated like a new one. Make sure the client receives a new analysis and consultation prior to any treatment being prescribed.

!
Health & Safety

Never apply a conditioning treatment to the scalp and hair if there is any sign of infection or infestation. (For further information see Chapter 15.)

4   During the combing process, ascertain the following: Is the hair dry and lacking moisture? Is the hair breaking? Is the hair discoloured? Is the scalp dry? Is the scalp dandruff infected/dry?

The following table can be helpful when selecting a suitable shampoo and conditioner.

Hair care problem	Recommended treatment	Result
Dandruff	Apply shampoo for dandruff (followed by a suitable conditioner depending on hair type)	Will control flaking/dandruff and irritation to the scalp.
Dry hair	Apply shampoo for dry hair	Will disentangle the hair and moisturise.
	Apply conditioning treatment for dry hair	Will add sheen and moisturise the scalp and hair.
Brittle/over-processed hair	Apply moisturising shampoo for brittle, damaged hair	Will disentangle the hair and moisturise.
	Apply restructurant conditioning treatment	Will add protein (amino acids) to the cortex of the hair; will control breakage/dryness and moisturise; will help to close the cuticle and make the hair appear smoother.

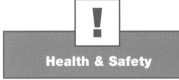

Health & Safety

Always make sure that all tools are clean and sterilised prior to use to avoid cross-infection.

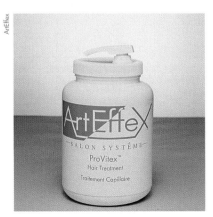

A conditioning product

Tools needed for a conditioning treatment

- large tooth comb
- bowl
- tinting brush
- towels
- plastic cape.

Application and removal of conditioning treatment

1   Prepare the client for the treatment by putting on the gown and towel.
2   Make sure conditioning treatment is applied to clean hair.
3   Section the hair into four by dividing from the front of the hairline to the nape and across the head from ear to ear (a).

Tip

Do not comb the hair prior to applying the conditioning treatment because this could cause breakage and damage to the hair.

Tip

Do not flood the hair with too much conditioner, as the hair can absorb only so much product. Excess product will be rinsed down the basin.

Tip

The use of additional heat will help to open the cuticle, allowing the conditioner to penetrate the hair.

4   Put the selected conditioning treatment in a bowl.

5   Take 6 mm (0.25 inch) sections, working from the nape upwards or the crown down to the nape. Using a tinting brush or cotton wool, start applying conditioner to the back sections first, working left to right (b). Proceed to the top sections, applying treatment to the left and then right section.

6   Work up or down the section, applying conditioner to the scalp and root area first. Once conditioner is applied thoroughly to this area, start applying conditioner to the middle lengths and ends (c).

7   After the application of conditioner, massage the scalp. (See Massage techniques.)

8   Apply heat using a steamer or dryer for approximately 10 minutes to half an hour. The more damaged the hair is, the longer the treatment will need to be left on.

Removal of conditioning treatment

The amount of rinsing that takes place will depend on the condition of the hair. On hair that is extremely damaged, it might be of greater benefit to the hair to leave some conditioner in and not to rinse all the product from the hair. However, when giving a normal treatment, rinse all the conditioner thoroughly from the hair.

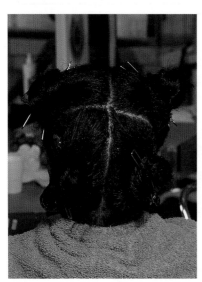

(a) Hair sectioned into four

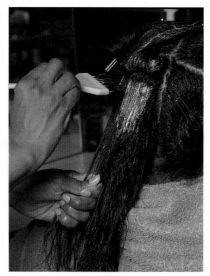

(b) Applying conditioner to the scalp and roots

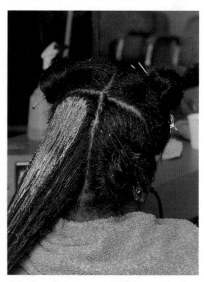

(c) Applying conditioner to the mid-lengths and ends

Massage techniques

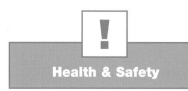

Make sure you wash your hands prior to giving a massage.

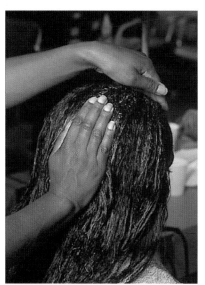

(a) Effleurage movement

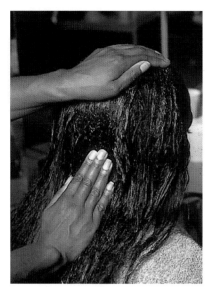

(b) Left hand following right hand, finishing the movement in the nape area

Scalp massage:

- stimulates the scalp by improving blood circulation
- increases oil production from the sebaceous glands
- breaks up fatty adhesions caused by blocked sebaceous glands
- helps stimulate hair growth
- relaxes the client.

Do not give a massage if any of the following contraindications are present:

- extreme pain, e.g. headache or migraine
- inflammation or broken skin
- contagious diseases such as ringworm, impetigo
- infestations such as lice and scabies.

As previously stated, the two movements used in massage are effleurage and petrissage.

- Effleurage is a gentle stroking movement that produces a soothing effect on the scalp.
- Petrissage is a kneading, lifting movement which stimulates the scalp and improves circulation to the veins and lymphatics.

A massage always starts and finishes with effleurage, with a period of petrissage in between. All massage movement must end in the nape area where the lymph glands are positioned.

Once the conditioning treatment has been applied, comb the hair from the ends, working up the mid-lengths to the roots in preparation for the massage.

Effleurage technique

1   Place both hands at the front hairline. Leading with the right hand and using the balls of the fingers, gently but firmly stroke the fingers downwards following the contours of the head (a). When your right hand reaches half way down the head, start stroking with the left hand starting at the front hairline. Finish the movement at the nape in the region of the lymph glands (b).

2   Continue with gentle but firm stroking movements, using alternate hands throughout. Work from the middle of the head to the left ear in continual stroking movements and back to the middle. Then work from the middle of the head towards the right ear (c).

Petrissage technique

1   Place both hands on the front hairline. Gently but firmly put pressure on the fingertips. Lift and knead the scalp between the fingertips.

2   Start the petrissage movement, working from the front of the head down to the nape (a).

3   Continue the petrissage movement, working from the middle of the head to the left ear in channels. Move from the left ear, working in channels from forehead to the nape across to the right ear (b).

4   Move from the right ear to the left ear and back to the right ear using the same technique as in 3.

5   If required, when the massage is complete, put a plastic cap on the head and apply additional heat if necessary (c).

6   Rinse the hair and finish as required.

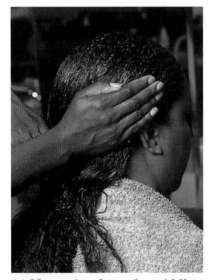

(c) Massaging from the middle of the head to the right ear

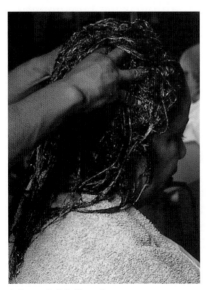
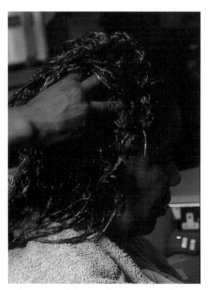
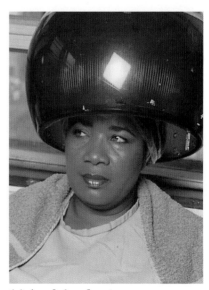

(a) and (b) Petrissage movement – lifting and kneading, working from the front hairline to the nape, and from ear to ear

(c) Applying heat

Setting

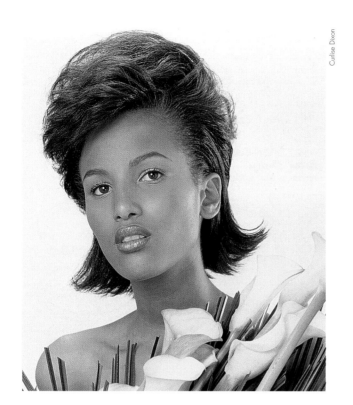

4

Curlise Dixon

Learning objectives

This chapter covers the following:

- **setting products and their use**
- **roller placement and selection**
- **consultation and analysis**
- **brick set**
- **directional set**
- **wrap set**
- **finger waves**
- **push waves**

Setting is a technique often used on African-Caribbean hair. The methods and techniques used are no different from setting Caucasian hair. A **cohesive set** is a temporary method of creating curl or movement in the hair and is best carried out on hair that has been chemically relaxed. African-Caribbean hair that has not been chemically relaxed can also be set so that the natural curl can be temporarily stretched to make the hair more manageable.

A cohesive set changes the keratin in the hair from **alpha keratin** to **beta keratin**. Alpha keratin exists when the hair is in its natural state, e.g. curly, wavy or straight. When the hair is set and dried on rollers or stretched during blow-drying, hydrogen bonds are temporarily broken and the hair takes on a new shape – the hair is now in a beta keratin state.

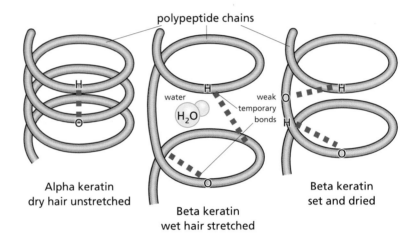

polypeptide chains

Alpha keratin
dry hair unstretched

water

weak
temporary
bonds

H_2O

Beta keratin
wet hair stretched

Beta keratin
set and dried

Once the hair has been blow-dried or set, it is in a temporarily stretched state. Being hygroscopic, the hair will gradually absorb moisture from the atmosphere and revert back to its former state. (For more information on alpha and beta keratin see the section on hair structure in Chapter 2.)

Setting products and their use

Setting products for African-Caribbean hair are designed to moisturise, protect the hair from the atmosphere and provide hold to preserve the finished look. Due to the dry nature of African-Caribbean hair, these setting products contain less alcohol and more conditioning agents than those used on Caucasian hair.

Alcohol has a drying effect when used on African-Caribbean hair. It is important not to dry the hair excessively. The setting lotions, gels or mousse used should therefore be specially formulated for African-Caribbean hair.

Types of setting products

The common setting products available are:

- **Setting lotions:** light conditioning lotions for blow-drying or setting styles which require a soft hold; firm hold products for waves, pincurls and sculptured looks.
- **Mousses:** used when a soft hold is required for setting and blow-drying the hair.
- **Gels:** used for styles requiring moulding, sculpturing or pincurling, especially when the hair needs to be set in a style where the finished look is solid and unmovable.

Setting products

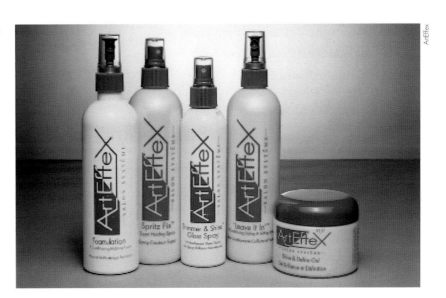

Roller placement and selection

Rollers can be placed in a variety of positions to create different effects, shapes and movement. Two basic principles must be followed if you are going to produce a good result when setting.

1 Sections taken prior to roller placement must not be wider or longer than the roller.
2 Each roller can sit on its own base to create volume and root movement. When using over-directed and under-directed techniques, each roller sits on one and a half times its own base so that volume is avoided at the root area.

Make sure the hair does not dry out during setting as this could cause the finished look to appear frizzy and dry instead of smooth. If the hair becomes dry while setting, keep it moist by spraying with water.

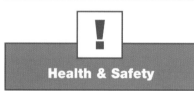

! Health & Safety

Make sure all tools are clean prior to setting. Dropped tools must be washed and sterilised before reusing.

Tip

Fish-hook ends will cause distorted and frizzy ends when combed out.

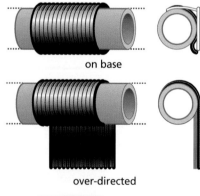

on base

over-directed

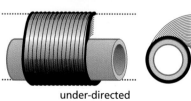

under-directed

3 When winding the hair on rollers, the hair should be wound around the roller at least one and a half times to ensure a uniformed curl is achieved.

Roller selection

The size of roller selected depends on the length of the hair, type of curl and movement desired.

- **Large rollers** will produce open, loose curls and create a softer, looser movement in the finished style; normally used on hair below the shoulder.
- **Medium rollers** will produce a firmer, tighter look and give the style more volume; normally used on hair just above the shoulder and shorter.
- **Small rollers** will produce tight curls and lots of volume – the finished style will be more durable; normally used on short hair or on medium to long hair where a curlier look is required.

Sectioning of the hair

Each section of hair taken prior to placing the roller must be cleanly combed to prevent distorted roots. The points of the hair must be curled evenly under the roller to avoid fish-hook ends.

There are three basic roller placements used when setting hair:

- **On-base roller:** This roller sits on its own base and creates volume, height and lots of root movement. This technique is ideal for styles that require a soft, full look and is one of the most commonly used techniques when setting hair.
- **Over-directed roller:** Used mainly on the front hairline to create straight, flat movement at the root, pushing the hair forward and producing volume on the ends. This technique is ideal for covering temples, particularly on styles where the hair has been designed to be styled away from the face.
- **Under-directed roller:** This technique tends to be used on the sides and back of the hair and keeps the hair at the roots in a flat position, avoiding the creation of any root lift or movement. When this technique of setting is used we often refer to the rollers as being 'dragged'. This is ideal for bobs and creating flatter, more head-hugging hairstyles.

Consultation and analysis

Tip

If even tension is not used, a frizzy, unstructured curl will result instead of a smoother, more structured curl.

Health & Safety

Avoid using undue tension when setting the hair particularly around the hair line, as this could cause traction alopecia. (For more information on traction alopecia see the section on hair loss in Chapter 15.)

When setting hair it is important to take into account a number of factors which will help you to achieve the desired finished look. When carrying out your consultation and analysis of the hair prior to setting, you need to assess the following areas:

- hair condition
- texture and density
- degree of natural curl
- nature of style to be achieved
- client's requirements
- setting product to be used.

It is important to conduct a detailed analysis and consultation as this will influence the final result and the durability of the style. When setting African-Caribbean hair it is important to keep the hair extremely smooth. Even tension must be used to avoid any distortion during the setting process.

Preparing the hair prior to setting

1 Analyse the hair texture, type and density to determine the correct roller placement and product selection for the look to be achieved and the durability of the hairstyle.
2 Discuss with your client the look to be created.
3 Shampoo and condition the hair in preparation for the set.
4 Comb the hair, making sure it is tangle free.
5 Apply the selected setting product to the hair.

Brick set

This technique of setting hair creates continual movement and allows the rollers to sit closer to each other, avoiding breaks/markation lines in the finished style.

To create a brick pattern set, rollers are placed like tiles on a roof.

Using this method to set the hair creates a much better finish and provides a continual line of movement in the dressed style. This is a much better option than channel

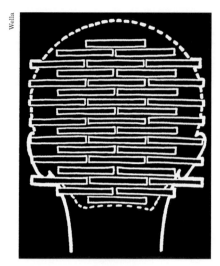

Rollers in brick pattern shape

Tip

Channel setting is a technique where the hair is set in rows throughout the head.

---

setting, which can produce breaks/markation lines in the finished hairstyle.

Follow steps 1 to 5 above for preparing the hair prior to setting, applying the appropriate setting/blow-dry lotion or mousse at step 5.

1 Comb the hair in the direction it is to be set. (For this style comb the hair to the side without a side parting.)

2 Take your first section of hair in the front hairline above the eyebrow. Place your first roller (a).

3 Place rollers behind the first roller in a brick fashion, working towards the ears. Wind the hair on the sides away from the face (b).

4 Take the next section of hair between each roller placed on the previous row.

5 Continue brick setting, following the same method of placing rollers in between each previous roller until the whole head is set (c).

6 Place the client under the dryer until the hair is completely dry.

7 Brush the hair thoroughly to remove markation lines.

8 Apply dressing or oil sheen spray if necessary to the scalp/ends of the hair.

9 Brush the hair into style; add height if required by back-combing the crown.

10 Apply finishing products as necessary (d) & (e).

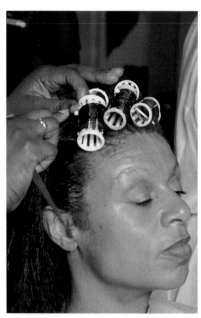

(a) Placing rollers on the hairline

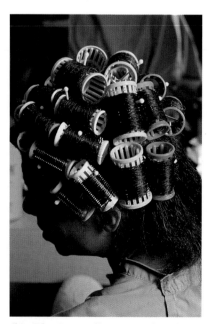

(b) Placing rollers in a brick pattern

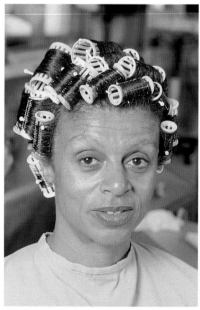

(c) The completed set

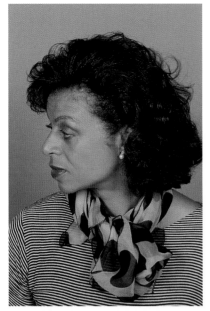

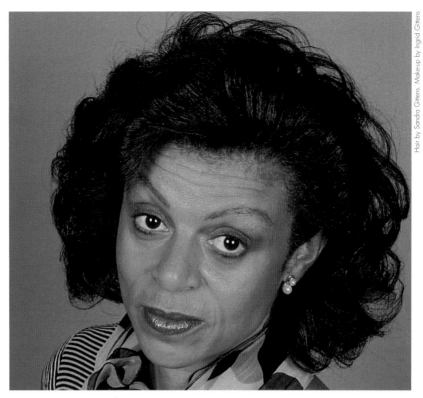

(d) & (e) The hair dressed out after the set – side (above); front (right)

11 Discuss with your client aftercare procedures and maintenance of the hairstyle. (For further information on aftercare see Chapter 6.)

Directional set

Tip

Combinations of setting techniques can be used to create a variety of looks.

This technique is used when you require the hair to be styled in a particular direction. The following are examples of directional sets:

- middle parting
- side parting
- flick up
- styled away from the face.

Follow steps 1 to 5 on page 49 for preparing the hair prior to setting, adding the appropriate setting/blow-dry lotion or mousse at step 5. The hair will be set with a middle parting and the hair flipped upwards on the perimeter. All rollers are placed in a brick fashion.

1 Part the hair in the middle. Place one roller on the crown (a).

2 Place rollers on each side of the parting in an under-directed position until you reach the ear, so that the hair is dragged to avoid root lift (b).

Tip

The arrows in the photographs show the direction the rollers have been placed in.

3   Continue to place another line of under-directed rollers behind the roller on the crown.

4   On the last three rows, wind the hair in an upward direction over the rollers. This will create a flick up when the hair is dry. Drag the root area to avoid root movement, keeping the hair smooth (c).

5   Place the client under the dryer until the hair is completely dry.

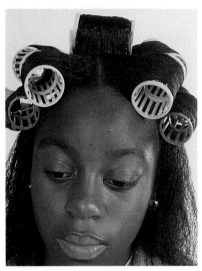 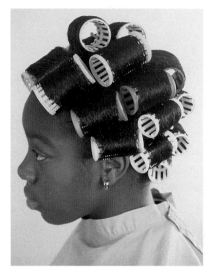 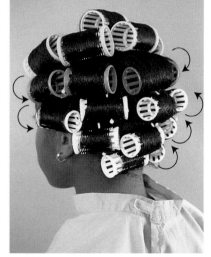

(a) & (b) One roller placed on the crown. Side rollers dragged to avoid root lift

(c) The last three rows are wound upwards

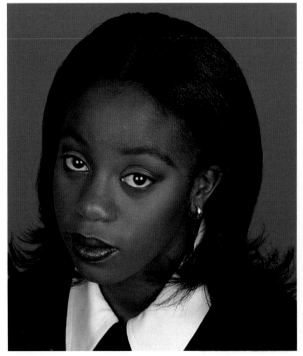 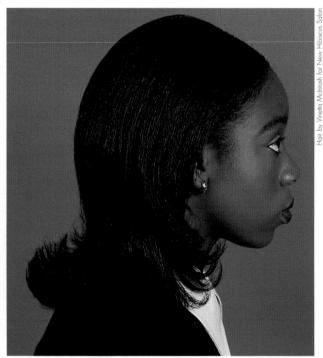

The finished style – front

The finished style – side

Hair by Vinetta McIntosh for New Hibiscus Salon

6   Brush the hair thoroughly to remove markation lines. Make sure you follow the direction the hair was set in when brushing, so that the shape is maintained.

7   Apply dressing or oil sheen spray if necessary to the scalp/ends of the hair.

8   Brush the hair into style; add height if required by back-combing the crown.

9   Apply finishing products as necessary.

10 Discuss with your client aftercare procedures and maintenance of the hairstyle. (For further information on aftercare see Chapter 6.)

Wrap set

Tip

Always keep the hair moist during wrap setting by spraying with water or lotion. Keeping the hair wet will make it more pliable and easier to mould close to the scalp.

A wrap set can be carried out on either short or long hair. This technique of setting produces a smooth look and uses the contours of the head to create shape and movement. Wrap setting provides a more natural form of setting without the tension which can be created by blow-drying and setting and is best used where a freer, smoother shape is required.

To add additional freedom and support after wrap setting, the hair can be blow-dried or tonged, or a combination of both techniques may be used to produce the finished hairstyle.

Wrap setting short hair

Follow steps 1 to 5 on page 49 for preparing the hair prior to setting, adding the appropriate blow-dry/wrap lotion or mousse at step 5.

1   Comb the hair thoroughly, starting from the nape and working up towards the front of the hairline.

2   Part the hair on the side (a).

3   Start by combing/brushing small sections of the hair flat against the scalp, working from the nape up to the crown (b).

4   Comb the hair on the opposite side of the parting, blending the hair away from the front hairline into the hair at the back of the head (c).

5   Comb the hair on the same side of the parting, close to the scalp and just over the hairline. Blend the hair at the side behind the ears into the back of the head and nape area. Keep the hair smooth and close to the head while wrapping.

6   Cover the hair with a net and dry under a hooded dryer.

7   When dry, brush the hair in the direction of the wrap to loosen the wrap set.

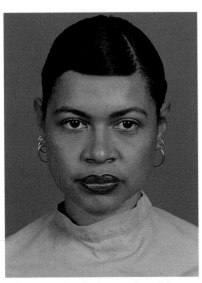

(a) **Part the hair on the side**

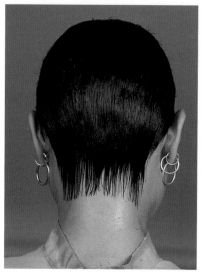

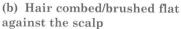

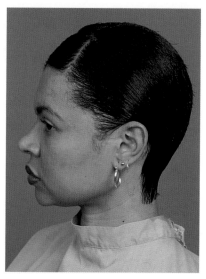

(b) Hair combed/brushed flat against the scalp

(c) Side hair blended into the back

Tip

When wrap setting, always mould the hair in the direction of the cut and finished style.

The finished hairstyle

8   Apply dressing or oil sheen spray to add sheen if required.

9   Finish the hair with a blow-dry. Tong the hair if additional support is required.

10 Apply finishing products.

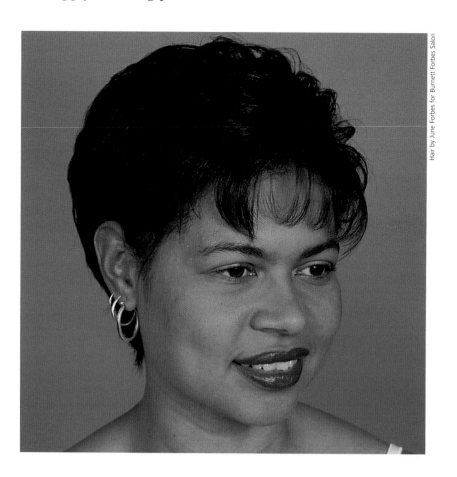

Hair by June Forbes for Burnett Forbes Salon

Wrap setting medium to long hair

Follow steps 1 to 5 on page 49 for preparing the hair prior to setting, applying the appropriate blow-dry/wrap lotion or mousse at step 5.

1 Place three rollers on the crown (on base) in a brick fashion (a).
2 Establish a side parting (b).
3 Take a small mesh of hair from the parting just under the rollers. Comb or brush the hair, keeping it close to the scalp (c).
4 Continue to blend the wrap by taking small meshes of hair and pivoting around the rollers in a spiral pattern, until the whole head is wrapped (d) & (e).

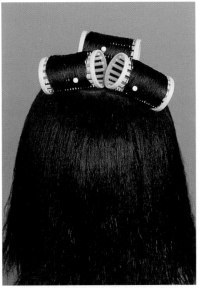

(a) Back showing three rollers on the crown

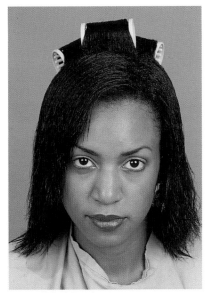

(b) Front showing side parting

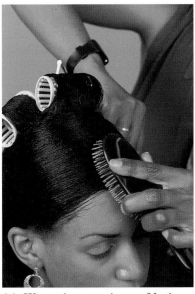

(c) Wrapping sections of hair from the parting

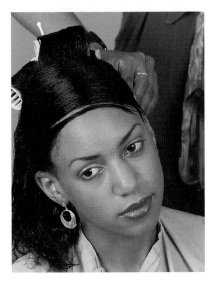

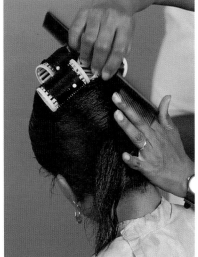

(d) & (e) Brushing and combing the hair around the head, keeping the hair smooth

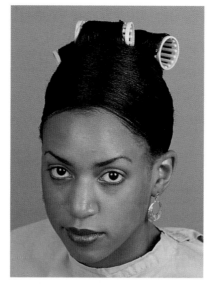
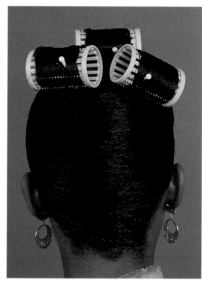

The finished wrap – front and back

Tip

Make sure the hair is thoroughly dry before attempting to comb it out. If it is still damp the curl will drop and the hair will become frizzy.

The finished look

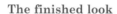

5   Place a net on the hair and put the client under the dryer. If the hair is long and thick, take the client out of the dryer after 20 minutes; reverse the wrap by combing

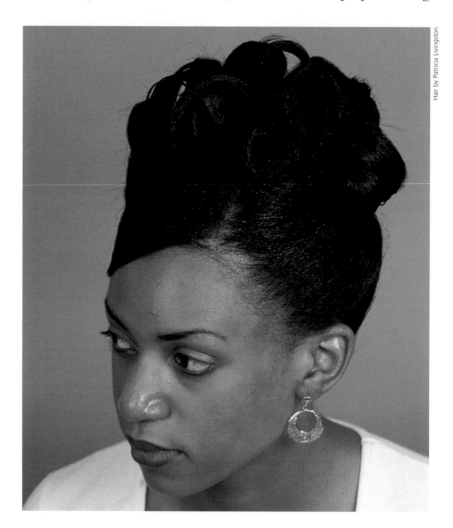

Hair by Patricia Livingston

the hair in the opposite direction and dry the hair for a further 15 to 20 minutes to make sure the underneath hair is dry.

6   Once the hair is dry, brush the hair out thoroughly.

7   Apply dressing or oil sheen spray if required.

8   Finish the hair with a blow-dry. Tong the hair if additional support is required.

9   Apply finishing products.

Finger waves

Finger waving is the moulding of the hair to produce solid waves throughout the head. This style is dependent on the use of strong setting gels or lotions which are specially designed for African-Caribbean hair. The products leave the hair with a solid finish once dry. Although these products have additional moisturisers built into them, continued use can have a drying effect on the scalp and hair. Because of the dry nature of this setting product, regular conditioning treatments must be recommended to the client to avoid the scalp and hair becoming dry.

Finger waves are made up of a crest and a trough movement. The crest is the raised part of the wave and the trough is the dip of the wave.

Follow steps 1 to 5 on page 49 for preparing the hair prior to setting, applying setting gel at step 5.

1   Comb the hair, starting from the nape and working up towards the front hairline to remove all tangles from the hair.

2   Using a styling comb, part the hair on the side.

3   Starting at the back, place the forefinger on the hair and comb the hair to the right (a).

4   Push the teeth of the comb to the right and upwards. Hold in position (a).

5   Replace the forefinger with the second finger and apply pressure, squeezing the crest of the wave between both fingers. Remove the comb (b).

6   Keep the fingers in position and comb the hair to the left (c).

7   Push the teeth of the comb to the left and upwards.

8   Move the second finger down onto the section of the hair you have just moulded.

9   Put the forefinger underneath as before and apply pressure, squeezing the wave between the fingers.

10   Continue using the same technique until the whole head is finger waved (d).

11   Place the client under the dryer. When the hair is completely dry, take the client out and apply oil and holding spray to the hair.

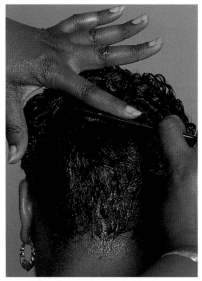

(a) Combing the hair to the right

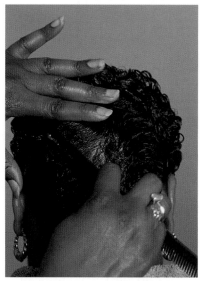

(b) Applying pressure and squeezing the wave with the fingers

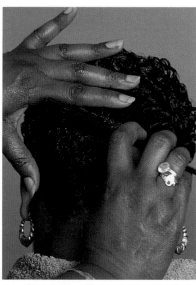

(c) Combing the hair to the left in preparation for the second finger wave

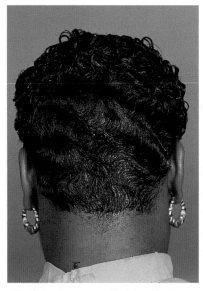

(d) Continue until the whole head is finger waved

Finished finger wave

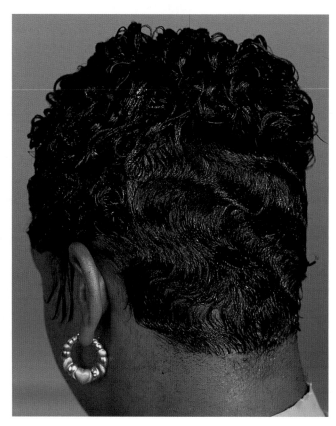

Push waves

This style is suitable for clients who require a look that is durable and needs little or no maintenance in between hairstyles. Push waves can be extremely drying to the scalp and hair because of the type of setting product used. When the hair is styled in this way it must be given conditioning treatments on a regular basis to moisturise the hair. Prolonged use of this technique to style the hair can cause breakage due to the drying effect of the setting products.

Follow steps 1 to 3 on page 49 for preparing the hair prior to setting.

Tip

The scalp must be kept moist by applying a suitable dressing prior to the setting product. Failure to apply dressing could result in a dry scalp and hair breakage.

Tip

To remove push waves from the hair, spray the hair with water until the hair is completely softened.

Tip

If you are still in training, you will need to practise under supervision before working on paying clients.

1   Comb the hair and apply a suitable dressing to the scalp.

2   Apply setting gel.

3   Comb the hair, starting from the nape and working up towards the crown and the front hair line.

4   Comb the hair and finger wave at least two rows across the front and sides.

5   Ensure the hair is combed flat against the head. Start push waves on the crown of the head. You will need two tail combs – one to hold the push wave in place and the other to disentangle the hair.

6   Comb the hair and lift with the end of the first tail comb. Do not remove the tail comb (a).

7   Hold the push wave firmly in place with the end of the second tail comb. Do not remove the comb (b).

8   Comb the hair to de-tangle (c).

9   Use the end of the first tail comb to disentangle the hair by sliding the tail comb through the underneath section of the hair (d).

10   Lift the push wave with the end of the first tail comb (e).

11   Hold the push wave in place with the end of the second tail comb (f).

12   Comb the hair and free the underneath hair with the first tail comb; lift the hair with the end of the tail comb.

13   Hold the push wave in place with the second tail comb.

14   Repeat the procedure until complete (g).

15   Fingerwave the hair at the back of the head.

16   Put the client under the dryer with a net for 15 minutes to partially dry the push wave movement into the hair. Remove the client from the dryer, lift the push wave into shape using the tail comb (h) & (i).

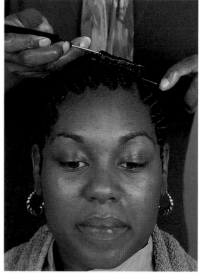

(a) Lifting the hair with a tail comb

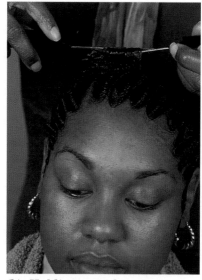

(b) Holding a push wave in place with a second tail comb

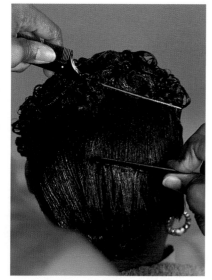

(c) Combing the hair to de-tangle

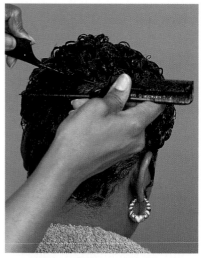

(d) Sliding the tail comb through a section of hair

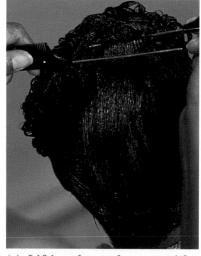

(e) Lifting the push wave with the end of the first tail comb

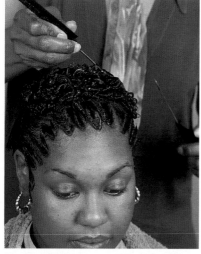

(f) Holding the push wave in place

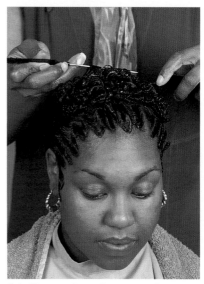

(g) Repeating the procedure until complete

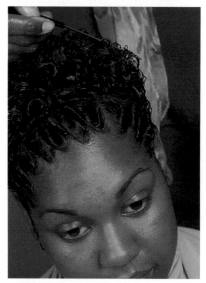

(h) & (i) Lifting the push waves into shape after removing the client from the dryer

The push waves must still be pliable enough to be lifted with the tail comb. If the hair is too dry, remoisten it lightly with blow-dry/wrap lotion. Replace the net on the hair and dry for another 20 minutes. When the hair is dry, spray with oil sheen spray and holding spray.

(For further information on the care of push waves see the section on aftercare in Chapter 6.)

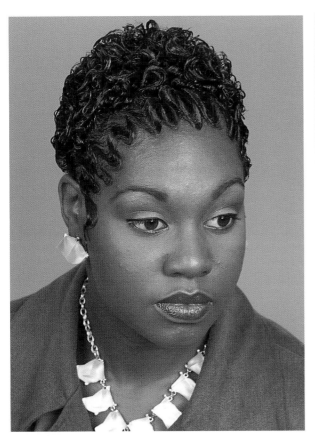 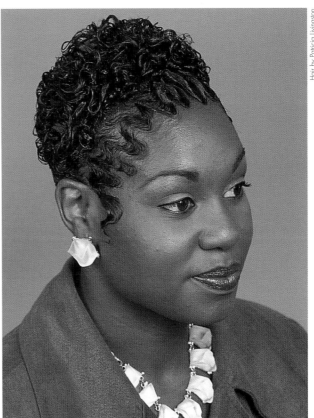

Hair by Patricia Livingston

The finished hairstyle – front and side

Blow-drying

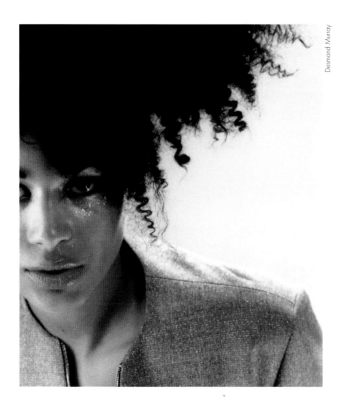

5

Desmond Murray

Learning objectives

This chapter covers the following:

- the correct use of blow-drying equipment
- blow-drying products and their use
- blow-drying using a comb attachment
- blow-drying using a comb or brush
- blow-drying using a spiral brush
- blow-drying after a set
- blow-drying after a wrap set
- scrunch drying

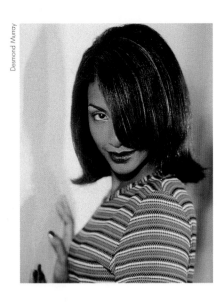

When blow-drying African-Caribbean hair, the same internal changes to the hair structure take place as when setting the hair. During the blow-drying process, the keratin of the hair is changed from alpha keratin to beta keratin, causing the hair temporarily to remain in its new shape. Once the hair takes in moisture from the atmosphere or becomes wet, it reverts back to its natural curl. (For further information see the sections on setting African-Caribbean hair in Chapter 4 and hair characteristics Chapter 2.)

Deciding which technique is to be used will depend on prior consultation and analysis with your client. Before attempting to blow-dry any head of hair you should consider the following:

- texture
- length
- condition
- desired finished look.

Once you have completed the consultation and analysis you will be able to decide on which blow-drying products and technique to use, and which tools you need to select to create the desired finished look. For example, using a spiral brush or blow-dry attachment.

A number of different blow-drying techniques can be used which will create movement and shape or a straight, smooth look. For example:

- A spiral brush will create curl and movement.
- A blow-drying attachment may be used to blow-dry the hair straight.
- Blow-drying the hair using a comb or brush will produce a straight effect.
- Blow-drying the hair after a set will loosen the curl and provide movement to the finished look.

You will need to know which of the above techniques to use to achieve the required look and shape, and whether the hair will also need to be tonged to provide additional support to the finished style.

The following **basic points** need to be observed prior to the blow-drying process:

- A thorough consultation and analysis must be made.
- Plan the direction and shape the hair is to be blow-dried in – the hair must be blow-dried in the direction the hair is to be styled.

- The client must be gowned and protected and the hair shampooed and conditioned.
- Blow-dry lotion or mousse must be used to protect the hair against the heat of the dryer.
- Wet hair must not be allowed to come into contact with hair already blow-dried.
- The blow-dryer must be kept moving to avoid burning the scalp and hair.
- Only blow-dry hair that is in good condition.

The correct use of blow-drying equipment

Correct care of equipment is important to avoid accidents while working in the salon. Before blow-drying any head of hair it is important to check that your blow-dryer is safe. Carry out the following checks prior to using a blow-dryer:

- Ensure that your hands are dry before touching the plug or switching on the dryer.
- Make sure the guard is securely placed so that the hair does not become entangled in the dryer.
- Ensure that the wires are not exposed and are fitted securely into the socket.
- Ensure that the hand dryer is in good working order by switching it on prior to use.

During use:

- Always switch off the hand dryer from the switch in the dryer and not from the socket.
- If the hand dryer starts to malfunction during use, turn the dryer off from the switch on the dryer and then the socket. Unplug the dryer from the socket.

After use:

- When you have finished using the blow-dryer, turn it off from the switch in the dryer first, then the socket. Pull the plug out of the socket.

Blow-drying products and their use

Products used to blow-dry African-Caribbean hair, like setting products, are designed to protect and moisturise the hair. Most blow-dry products have light conditioning properties built into them and contain little or no alcohol. They are mainly of two types, **lotions** and **mousses**, although **cream-based** products have recently been added to the range.

Blow-dry lotion

Blow-dry lotion is in the form of a spray with little or no holding properties so that the hair remains pliable, allowing the use of blow-dry brushes or an attachment. The non-addition of alcohol will avoid the hair becoming too dry and breaking. This product is best used on the following types of hair:

- hair that requires a soft, flexible finish
- hair that has recently been chemically processed
- damaged, dry, brittle hair.

Mousse

Two types of mousse are suitable for blow-drying African-Caribbean hair. The first type contains a small amount of alcohol and polyquaternium to help retain curl and the finished style. This type of mousse is best used on hair which is not dry and is in good condition. The second type of mousse contains no alcohol or polyquaternium, but adds moisture and sheen to the hair. This product is suitable for natural, permed and relaxed hair which is in good condition.

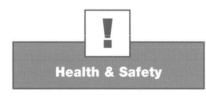

Health & Safety

Always make sure your hands are dry prior to holding a hairdryer to avoid electric shocks.

Blow-dry cream

Blow-dry creams coat the hair, which helps to moisturise it and gives it a silky appearance. They are best suited to:

- short hair
- wrap setting prior to blow-drying
- dry/damaged hair in need of moisture
- naturally curly hair

Preparing the client and hair prior to blow-drying

1   Gown the client.
2   Carry out a consultation and analysis of the hair.
3   Think about the hair type, product and technique to be used.

4   Provide the client with feedback on how the hair is to be blow-dried and the effect to be achieved.

5   Shampoo and condition the hair.

6   Comb the hair to remove any tangles and apply blow-drying product.

Blow-drying using a comb attachment

Tip

When you become proficient at blow-drying you can use fewer sections or no sectioning at all.

This technique is ideal for creating smoother, straighter looks and can be used either on hair that has been relaxed or hair that is still in its natural form. See Chapter 13 on natural hair.

Follow steps 1 to 6 above for preparing the client and hair prior to blow-drying.

Technique

1   Attach the comb attachment to the blow-dryer.

2   Section the hair into four.

3   Sub-divide the hair, working from the nape section, sectioning the hair from left to right.

4   Comb each section thoroughly.

5   Hold the blow-dryer by the handle for control.

6   Slide the comb attachment through the hair slowly, starting from the middle back section. Working from left to right, begin at the ends and work up through the middle lengths to the roots (a), (b) & (c).

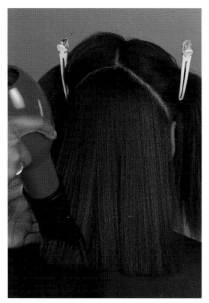

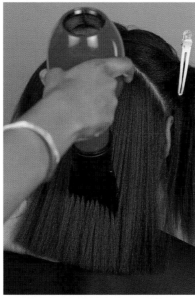

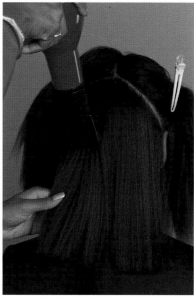

(a) Blow-drying using the comb attachment on the ends of the hair

(b) Blow-drying the middle lengths

(c) Blow-drying the roots

Tip

When blow-drying it is important to be consistent, drying the hair methodically to avoid leaving sections either still wet or under/over dried. This could cause an uneven texture in the finished result.

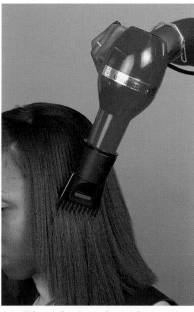

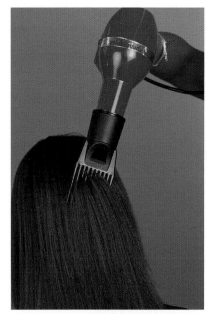

(d) Blow-drying the crown area   **(e) Blow-drying the side section**

The finished blow-dry

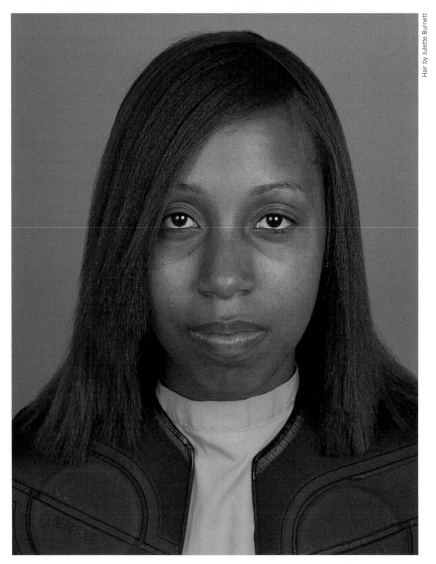

Hair by Juliette Burnett

Tip

It is better to blow-dry African-Caribbean hair using the full heat and power of the dryer. This will result in a smoother finish. Blow-dry product must be used to minimise damage to the hair.

7   Repeat the process until the hair in that section is completely dry and straight.

8   Continue to work up to the crown of the head until you reach the horseshoe section (d).

9   Start blow-drying the side section by sub-dividing the hair in 6 mm (0.25 inch) sections (e).

10   Work up the head until you reach the horseshoe section.

11   Repeat the process on the other side of the head.

12   Start blow-drying the horseshoe section using the same technique as before, working through to the front hairline. Blow-dry the hair in the direction it is to be styled. If the hair needs to be straighter repeat the process, working up through the nape area to the front hairline taking 6 mm sections throughout the hair. The finished effect is smooth and straight, ideal for one-length bobs and for styles that require little or no movement. The hair can be tonged after blow-drying if more movement and direction is required.

Blow-drying using a comb or brush

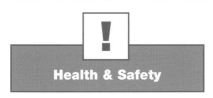

Health & Safety

Keep the blow-dryer moving constantly to avoid burning the scalp and hair.

Using a comb or brush to apply tension to the hair, followed by the blow-dryer, will produce a similar effect to blow-drying with a comb attachment.

Technique

Follow steps 1 to 6 on page 66–7 for preparing the client and hair prior to blow-drying.

1   Follow steps 2 to 5 of the previous technique.

2   Attach the blow-dry nozzle to the hairdryer so that the air will be concentrated on the area you are blow-drying.

3   Start to blow-dry from the nape section.

4   Using a comb or brush, comb the hair, applying tension with the comb followed by the blow-dryer.

5   Once one section is dry, proceed to another section.

6   Keep the hair in a smooth state while blow-drying so that kinks do not appear in the finished style.

7   Continue to blow-dry the hair, working through the sections until you get to the front hairline.

8   Change direction by blow-drying the hair around the front hairline in a backward movement away from the hairline. This will ensure that the whole head is blow-dried to the same degree.

9   The hair can be tonged if more movement, direction and a straighter look are required.

Blow-drying using a spiral brush

Tip

Make sure the hair is completely dry before proceeding to a new section of hair.

Tip

Remember to blow-dry the hair in the direction it is required to lie. For example, if you blow-dry the hair upwards the hair will move in an upward direction; sideways and the hair will move towards the side.

The purpose of using this technique is to straighten and dry the hair while adding curl and movement. It is best used on hair that has been cut in a suitable style, for example a one-length, graduated, or layered cut.

Technique

Follow steps 1 to 6 on page 66–7 for preparing the client and hair prior to blow-drying. Select a suitable size brush depending on the length of the hair, the style to be achieved and the requirements of the client.

1   Section the hair into four.
2   Sub-divide the hair from ear to ear, starting at the nape.
3   Start blow-drying the hair from the nape area, working from the middle then the left and right sections. Take meshes no more than 6 mm (0.25 inches) in width (a).
4   Place the blow-dry brush under the section to be blow-dried.
5   Apply heat to the root area first and gently pull the brush through the hair, followed by the hairdryer. Proceed onto the mid-lengths and then the ends. Continue with this technique until the hair in this section is completely dry.
6   Apply the same technique to both sides of the hair (b).
7   Continue blow-drying the crown and the fringe area of the hair into the style and shape required (c).

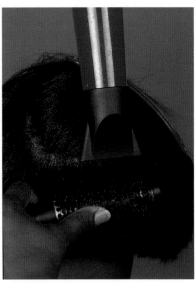

(a) Blow-drying the nape area

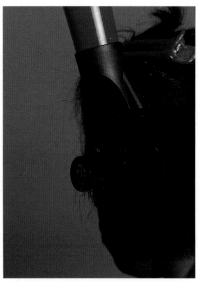

(b) Blow-drying the sides

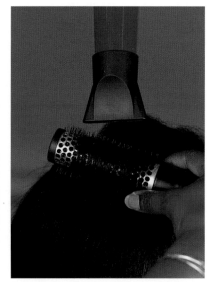

(c) Blow-drying the crown

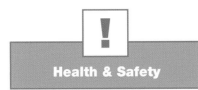

8   If you require more movement and shape, when the hair is dry wind the hair around the brush and apply heat by using the blow-dryer to the curled hair. Remove the blow-dryer and let the hair cool before unwinding the brush. This process will create more movement in the hair and add length and durability to the blow-dry and the finished style. Tonging the hair after blow-drying will add additional support.

9   Apply finishing products.

The finished look

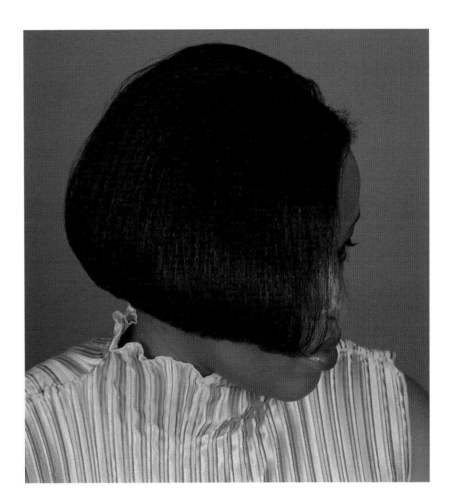

Blow-drying after a set

The purpose of blow-drying after a set is to create a smoother, softer movement to the finished look. This technique is suitable for dry, damaged hair or for hair which has just been relaxed and needs to be treated gently, but still requires a softer movement. Hair that is natural and has been set is ideal to blow-dry after setting.

Tip

Over-application of hair dressing or oil spray will cause the hair to become lank and detract from the finished style.

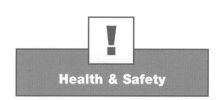

Although blow-drying hair that is already dry is kinder to the hair, excessive heat can cause the scalp and hair to become dry and damaged; in extreme cases the scalp and hair can be burnt. Take care therefore when blow-drying wet or dry hair.

The blow-drying technique will stretch the hair and smooth the cuticle in preparation for tonging.

Technique

1   After setting and drying, remove the rollers and brush the hair out thoroughly to remove markation lines.

2   Apply hair dressing sparingly to the scalp and hair if necessary. Oil sheen spray can be used if preferred.

3   Start blow-drying the hair from the nape, then the middle section, working left to right as in the previous technique.

4   Continue working up the head towards the front hairline.

5   Blow-dry the roots, mid-lengths and then the ends, until the hair is completely smooth.

6   When the whole mesh of hair is smooth, roll the hair onto a brush and apply heat. Leave the hair to cool for a few seconds. This technique will produce a smooth finish, as well as a strong curl and movement within the finished style.

Blow-drying after a wrap set

The purpose of blow-drying the hair after a wrap set is to encourage greater flexibility, definition, direction and movement within the finished style. The hair can be tonged if additional support and direction is required. This technique is suitable for all hair types, but should only be used when you want to achieve a straighter, softer look.

Technique

1   Brush the hair out thoroughly in the direction of the wrap set.

2   Apply hair dressing oil sheen to the scalp and hair sparingly if required.

3   Select which brush is to be used – spiral or Denman. The type of brush selected will depend on the shape, movement and style required:

● For styles requiring more movement and body select a spiral brush.

● For straighter looks use a Denman brush.

4 Start by blow-drying the hair from the nape, working upwards (a).

5 Continue blow-drying the hair following the direction of the wrap set (b).

6 Use this technique to blow-dry the hair, progressing throughout the crown towards the front hairline (c).

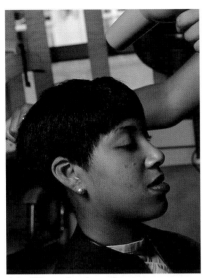 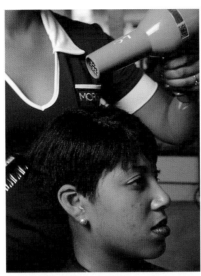 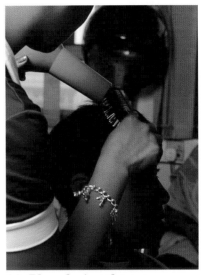

(a) Blow-drying the nape area

(b) Blow-drying the hair in the direction of the set

(c) Blow-drying the crown

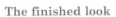The finished look

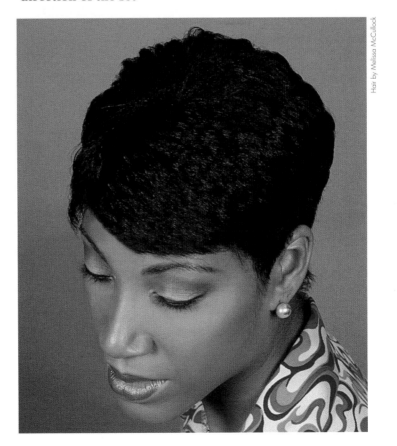

Hair by Melissa McCullock

Scrunch drying

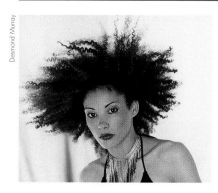

Desmond Murray

This technique can be used on African-Caribbean hair that is naturally curly or wavy, or on hair that has been permed. It is particularly suitable for hair that has been body waved. Scrunch drying will help expand the curl, giving definition and separation to the finished style.

Technique

Shampoo and condition the hair before blow-drying. Comb the hair out thoroughly and apply a suitable activator and moisturiser for permed or naturally curly hair.

1   Attach a diffuser to the blow-dryer.
2   Apply medium heat and air flow to the hair. Scrunch the hair between your fingers, cupping the hair in your hand to support the curl (a).
3   Apply the diffuser to the hair and hold, pushing against the curl. This will help maintain the curl formation (b).

Tip

Over-drying the hair when scrunch drying could cause the hair to become frizzy. To keep curl separation, some moisture should be left within the hair. For maximum effect leave the hair semi-dry. If the hair becomes too dry, moisturise with an oil sheen spray or activator.

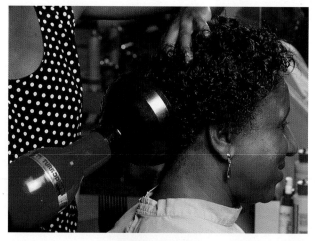

(a) Scrunching and drying with the diffuser

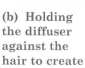

Health & Safety

Make sure the diffuser and hairdryer are not held in one position for too long. This could over-dry the hair and cause damage to the hair and scalp.

(b) Holding the diffuser against the hair to create definition

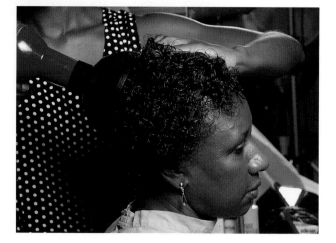

4   Use this technique throughout the scrunch dry, working from the nape to the crown and front hairline (c).

5   Apply additional mousse or oil sheen spray if the hair has become over dry. Holding spray can be added to create direction, hold and separation to the finished style.

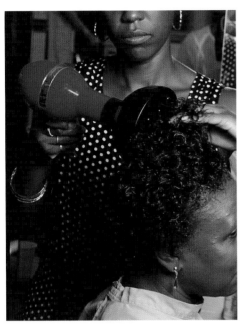

(c) Blow-drying the crown, lifting the hair to create height

The finished scrunch dry

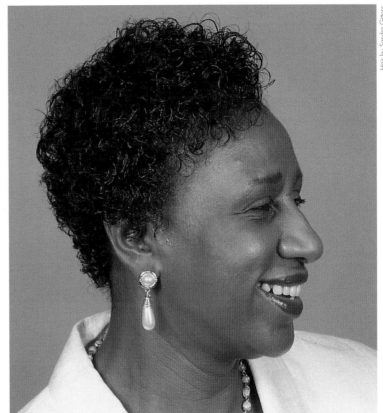

Hair by Sandra Gittens

Styling and finishing

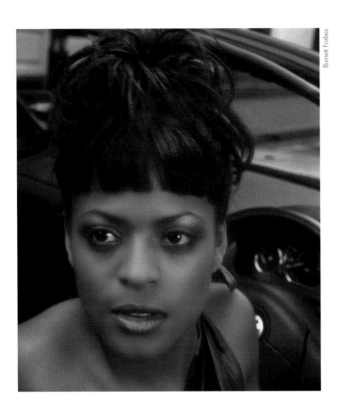

Burnett Forbes

Learning objectives

This chapter covers the following:

- face shapes
- styling tools
- finishing products and their use
- styling techniques
- client aftercare

6

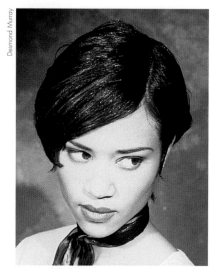

Commercial

Creating the finished look is important when styling the hair. The style must enhance the client's features and personality. To enable you to do this, several points need to be taken into consideration before proceeding to style the hair:

- client's lifestyle
- client's face shape
- any chemical process that has been applied to the hair
- the style the hair was set or blow-dried in
- the occasion the hair is being styled for
- balance and shape to be achieved
- the tools needed to style the hair
- maintenance and aftercare.

Different images can be created when styling the hair. Hairstyles fall into the following categories:

- **Commercial look** – an everyday look that is suitable for a variety of people and is easy to wear.
- **Fashion look** – a style that is currently in fashion and worn for a period or until it is no longer fashionable.
- **Classic look** – a style that never dates or goes out of fashion, for example a bob.
- **Avant-garde look** – a style that is ahead of its time; usually worn by the leaders of fashion before the look becomes fashionable.

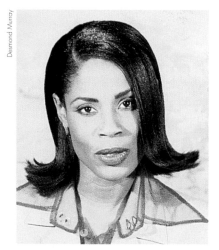

Fashion

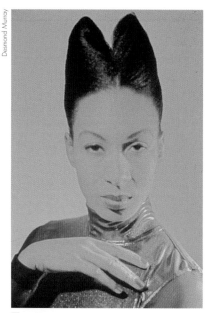

Fantasy

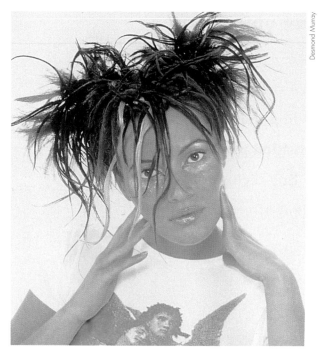

Avant-garde

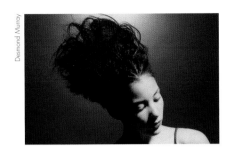

- **Fantasy look** – usually seen in competition hairstyling; not worn as an everyday style; the look is very dressed and exaggerated.

An understanding of how looks are interpreted, created and achieved is important. These factors need to be taken into consideration before you can start creating and designing a suitable hairstyle, haircut, blow-dry or set for your client.

Face shapes

Tip

To determine your client's face shape, comb the hair away from the scalp; put the hair in a pony tail if long enough. For shorter hair use a bandeau – this will enable you to see the shape of the face clearly.

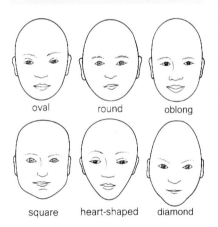

oval round oblong

square heart-shaped diamond

When you create a hairstyle for a client, the face shape and any prominent features such as a large nose or protruding ears must be also be taken into consideration. Years ago, hairdressers had preconceived ideas about which styles were suitable for certain face types. Over the years there has been a change in thinking regarding styles that can and cannot be worn. Many stylists believe and work with the concept that any style can be worn by any face shape so long as it is tailored to suit the client's features and personality.

The completed style must not draw attention to any irregularities in the face shape but rather distract from them. For example, a client with a full face should not have width on the side of the face or a full heavy fringe as these would make the face appear wider. To complement a full face, the hair could be styled forward with wispier sides and fringe. The rest of the hair could be styled to the side or away from the face with height on the crown.

The perfect face shape is supposed to be oval because there are no irregular contours. When you style the hair you are trying to create the correct balance and shape for the face and in some respects achieve the perfect face shape.

The table outlines the six different face shapes with styling tips.

Face shape	Styling tips
Oval	Can wear any style
Round	Needs height and not too much width on the sides; length can be left at the nape
Square	Needs a style to counteract the angular shape and create softness and roundness, possibly covering the jawbone; side partings can help detract from squareness
Oblong	Requires fullness to add width; no height needed; a fringe can be added to shorten the face
Heart-shaped	Needs a style that will be narrow at the temples and wider at the chin
Diamond	Needs width at the temple and jaw or chin

Prominent features on the face also need to be taken into consideration when styling the hair. Several examples are described in the following table.

Prominent feature	Unsuitable hair style	Suitable hair style
Protruding ears	Hair combed behind the ears	Hair styled to cover the ears
High forehead	Hair swept away from the forehead	A full fringe or half fringe to soften the forehead
Receding chin	Hair swept back from the face; height on the crown	Side parting combined with fullness at the nape
Protruding chin	Hair styled away from the chin	A style that covers the jaw line avoiding sharp lines; round shapes to create softness

Tip

It is important that you use tact and show sensitivity towards the client at all times to avoid causing offence.

As a hair-stylist it is important that you do not draw your client's attention to any prominent features but mentally make a note of them and style the hair in such a way that it diverts attention away from them.

Some clients are extremely conscious of their looks and will confide in you their concerns. Always try to reassure clients and build their confidence. Never openly agree with them.

Tip

Middle partings are the most difficult to create as they can easily become crooked. The following technique can be used to create a balanced centre parting:

● Comb the hair back away from the face.

● Using the tip of the comb, lightly draw it along the bottom centre of the nose until you reach the hairline.

● Use the point of the comb to draw a line through the hair and establish a middle parting.

Partings

Partings can create all sorts of illusions, some of which can be unflattering:

● A wide parting can cause the client's face to appear too wide and flat.

● On the wrong client a middle parting can make the face appear too wide, drawing attention to other features on the face.

● Partings which are too long could cause the crown to appear flat and the hair to lack height in this area.

● If you are creating a straight parting, ensure that it *is* straight.

The following partings can be used to create diversity in a hairstyle:

● Zig-zag partings can create interest to the finished style. These partings work well if combined with styles that are not too fussy.

● Asymmetric partings can create interest and variety to a hairstyle.

Styling tools

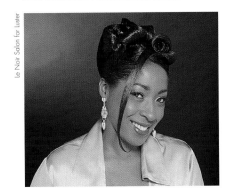

Le Noir Salon for Luster

A variety of tools can be used to style the hair and create different effects.

- **Afro comb:** used to style natural afro hairstyles or to lift hairstyles. This is ideal for curly hair.
- **Styling combs:** suitable for combing the hair out after a set, blow-dry or wrap set. These come in a variety of sizes – use a size you are comfortable with. The closer set teeth are used for back-combing/teasing the hair; the larger teeth are used to smooth the hair after back-combing or to style and dress the hair.
- **Rake comb:** ideal for creating separation and breaking up solid styles.
- **Back-combing comb:** ideal when back-combing – the pick is used for lifting the hair to create height.
- **Paddle brush:** used to brush the hair out after a set, blow-dry, wrap set. Ideal for keeping the hair smooth and flat.
- **Bristle brush:** used in the same way as the above.
- **Denman brush:** used in the same way as the above.
- **Vent brush:** used to create spiky, tousled looks.

Tip

The tools you use should be sterilised after each client to avoid cross-infection. (For information on sterilising tools see Chapter 15.)

Finishing products and their use

Tip

Be careful how you apply dressings when dealing with very fine hair as they could cause the hair to lose body and become lank and difficult to style. Oil sheen spray can be used in place of a dressing cream if the hair is fine or you require a lighter product.

Products go a long way towards helping the stylist create the finished look. It is important, therefore, that you have a good knowledge of finishing products and their uses. This will help you to achieve the best results and enable you to advise your clients on aftercare. Different products will help you achieve a variety of results:

- **Hairdressing creams** can be heavy or light in consistency. The selection of a dressing will depend on the hair texture, for example coarse textured hair will require a heavier dressing and more product; fine textured hair will need a lighter dressing and less product. Dressing should be applied sparingly to avoid flooding the scalp and hair. Only use a dressing if the scalp or ends of the hair are dry.
- **Oil sheen spray** can be used as an alternative to dressings. It is less oily and is absorbed easily by the hair, so is ideal for fine, lank hair. Oil sheen spray can also be used to give added shine to the hair after

Tip

On permed hair, failure to use finishing products could cause the hair to become dry, frizzy and brittle. Finishing products also need to be used on natural hair to make the hair easier to comb out and give the hair shine. (It is not crucial that activator is applied to natural hair.)

using a dressing. It is suitable for both relaxed and permed hair.

- **Gel** can be used on relaxed or permed hair during styling to keep the hair flat and neat on the sides and the back. It is also suitable for upswept hair styles to control stray hair. Avoid using alcohol-based gels on permed hair as they can make the hair dry.

- **Holding spray** is used after styling relaxed hair to hold it in place. Holding sprays come in light or strong hold formulas. Selection of the product will depend on how the hair is styled and durability required. For example, styles which need to be more mobile would be better suited to a light hold spray whereas a hairstyle that needs to be much firmer will require a stronger hold.

- **Spritz** is a firm hold spray used where a solid hold is required. It is ideal for upswept, scrunch or freeze styles on naturally curly or relaxed hair. It provides sheen to the hair and an immovable finish.

- **Hair moisturiser** is suitable for permed or natural hair. It comes in the form of a spray and coats the hair, making it easier to comb. It also adds sheen to the hair.

- **Activator** gives definition to permed or naturally curly hair. It increases the curl, adds control and stops the hair becoming frizzy. It conditions the hair and makes the hair pliable.

- **Moisturiser/activator** is a combined product which avoids the use of two products, making application easier. It is suitable for permed and natural hair, and works well on dry hair.

- **Serum** is used where maximum shine is required. It has no holding properties and is ideal for use on relaxed hair. It will give definition to the finished style.

Application of dressing

1 Comb the hair through, starting from the nape up to the hairline.
2 Part the hair down the middle and lightly apply dressing to the scalp (a).
3 Starting at the nape, section the hair using a comb (b).
4 Apply dressing to the scalp, working up to the front hairline (c) & (d). Massage the dressing into the scalp.
5 Rub the dressing into the ends of the hair (e).

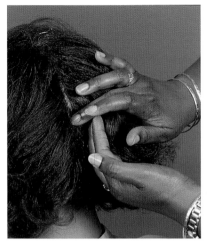

(a) Applying dressing to the scalp using a central parting

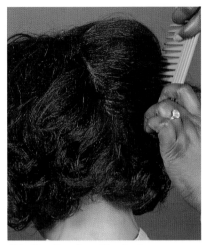

(b) Sectioning the hair

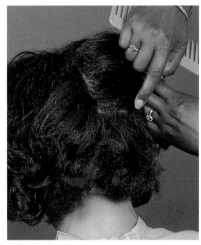

(c) Applying dressing to the scalp

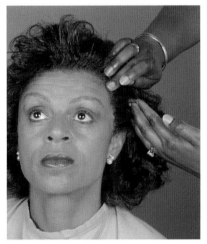

(d) Applying dressing to the front hairline

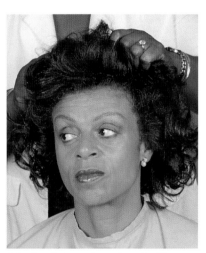

(e) Applying dressing to the ends

The finished hair style after dressing has been applied

Tip

Oil sheen spray can be used in place of a dressing, following the technique above.

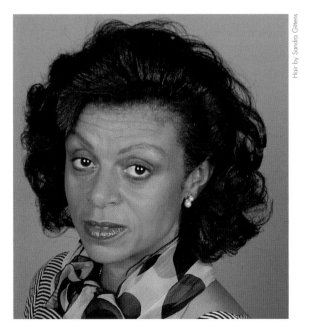

Hair by Sandra Gittens

Styling techniques

Tip

When a hairstyle comes back into fashion it is always slightly different from the original look. Hairstyles are influenced by current fashion and social trends.

As discussed at the beginning of this chapter (page 78), several factors need to be considered when creating a hairstyle. Chapter 10 discusses how hairstyles and fashion revolve. As a student of hairdressing, you need to learn basic skills which are relevant to all styles, so that when styles become fashionable again you will know how to achieve them.

As a stylist it is important to keep up to date with the latest fashion in hair, clothes and make-up. This can be achieved by observing looks seen on the street, in clubs, at fashion shows, in fashion magazines, television pop videos and technical videos.

Tip

Once you have learnt the basics of hairdressing thoroughly, you can progress to more advanced hairstyling techniques.

Back-combing/back-brushing

Creating height can play an important part in developing the finished style. This can be achieved by using one of the two following techniques:

- back-combing
- back-brushing.

These techniques involve brushing or combing the hair through after setting/wrap-setting, blow-drying or tonging. The following method can be used for either back-combing or back-brushing.

Tip

Always back-comb the hair at the back of the section and not the front, as this could cause a ruffled appearance, making it difficult to create a smooth finish.

Tip

Using the large side of the comb will produce body and volume in the finished style; the finer side of the comb will produce a solid, immovable finish. Selecting which side of the comb to be used will depend on the look you want to achieve.

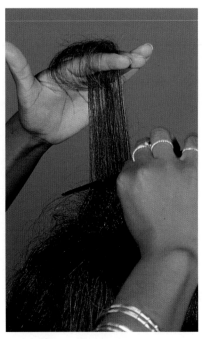

Back-combing the hair

1   Take a section of hair no wider than 6 mm (0.25 inches).

2   With one hand, hold the hair firmly in an upward position between the fingers.

3   With the other hand hold the comb between the thumb and fingers.

4   Place the teeth of the comb at the back of the section, 6 mm away from the scalp.

5   Push the teeth of the comb downwards towards the scalp.

6   Place the comb above the section you have just

Tip

You can back-comb a strand of hair so that it will be solid from roots to points. Only put as much back-combing in the hair as required to achieve the hairstyle. If 25 mm (1 inch) of back-combing/brushing is required, do not back-comb the hair more than is necessary. To remove back-combing/-brushing, comb or brush the hair gently from the ends, working up to the roots.

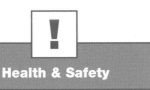

Health & Safety

Always back-comb or back-brush the hair gently to avoid breaking the hair or splitting the cuticle. For more information on hair structure see the relevant section in Chapter 2.

Tip

Only porous hair or hair that has a variety of different lengths will hold back-combing. Hair in good condition or all the same length will be difficult to back-comb.

back-combed. Using the same technique as before, gently push the hair down on top of the previous section. Continue to build on the back-combing in this way until the required height and width is achieved.

7 Comb the hair on the outer side of the back-combing to create a smooth finish.

Styling the hair after a directional or brick set

1 Brush out the hair thoroughly, starting from the nape and working up the hair to the front hairline.

2 Brush the hair in the direction it was set to blend in the roller markations.

3 Apply dressing or oil sheen spray to the hair as required.

4 If additional height is required add back-combing or back-brushing, dressing the hair from the nape and working upwards.

5 Look critically at the balance, shape, style and movement being created.

6 Adjust the height if required by lifting with a tail comb or styling pick. At this stage you should be looking at the face shape and taking the client's requirements into account to ensure the hairstyle created suits the customer.

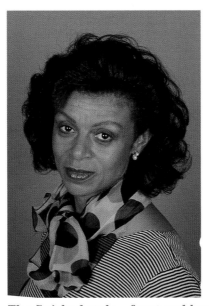
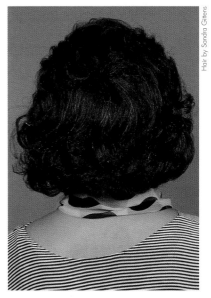

The finished style – front and back

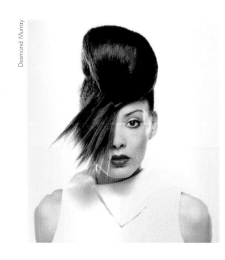

Desmond Murray

Styling the hair after a wrap set

This method can be used to style the hair after wrap-setting using the round brush technique.

1 Brush out the hair thoroughly, following the direction of the wrap set (see Chapter 4).
2 Apply dressing or oil sheen spray sparingly to avoid the hair becoming limp during blow-drying.
3 Blow-dry the hair to create smoothness, movement and mobility if required.
4 The hair can be tonged if more support is needed.
5 Dress the hair in the desired style. Apply oil sheen or holding spray if required.

Finishing the hair after finger-waving or push-waving

1 Once the hair has been thoroughly dried, apply oil sheen spray; use holding spray to give additional support if required.(For further information see Chapter 4.)

Styling the hair after scrunch drying

This technique can be used to finish the hair after a perm or on naturally wavy hair (see Chapter 5).

1 Use activator mousse to create separation and add moisture if the hair has been over-dried.
2 Spray on moisturiser to add shine to the hair.
3 Style the hair using a pick or styling comb according to the client's requirements and the shape of the cut.

Styling permed hair

This method is used on permed hair and is also suitable for clients who have naturally curly or wavy hair.

1 After the hair has been permed or shampooed and conditioned, towel dry.
2 Pour activator or wave lotion into the palm of the hand (a).
3 Apply activator or wave lotion to the scalp by taking 6 mm (0.25 inch) sections (b).
4 Apply additional product to the mid-lengths and ends of the hair and massage the scalp (c).
5 Apply moisturising spray (d).

6 The client can be put under a cool dryer till the hair is semi-dry or alternatively the scrunch dry method can be used to finish the hair.

7 Apply activator mousse or activator, wave lotion and moisturising spray to create separation and definition to the curl.

8 Finish the hair, taking into account the client's requirements, face shape and haircut. Use a pick or comb to style the hair.

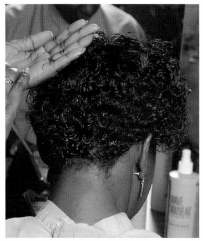

(a) Activator in the palm of the hand

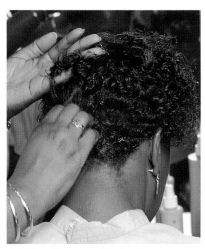

(b) Sectioning the hair and applying activator to the scalp

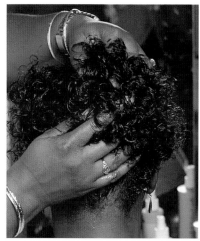

(c) Applying activator to the ends

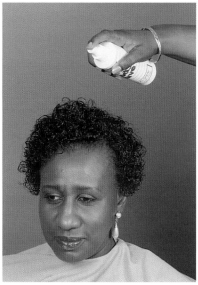

(d) Applying moisturising spray

The finished style after applying oil sheen spray

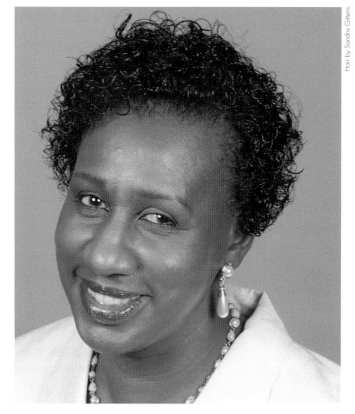

Hair by Sandra Gittens

Tip

A French plait can be styled to the right or left of the head. If you are right-handed your plait should be coiled to the right and vice versa if you are left-handed.

Tip

For a smoother, flatter French plait, do not add back-combing

Tip

Using the overlapping technique when placing grips in the hair will avoid the hair slipping out from the clipped area.

Tip

Always apply oil sheen spray first rather than last. Using holding spray first will protect the hair and form a barrier to the oil sheen spray.

Styling techniques for long hair

The styling of long hair is a specialist area that can provide a platform for the stylist to be creative. A client with long hair has the option of a variety of styles. Any styling work on long hair should be neat and tidy with all pins and clips hidden.

The following hairstyles can be used on hair that is shoulder length and longer:

French plait

This style can be achieved on pre-set or un-set hair. It is ideal for weddings, parties and any formal occasion. A French plait can be styled with several options, for example a side or middle parting, swept back away from the face. The direction in which the front of the hair is to be styled is also optional and will depend on the occasion, face shape client's requirements.

Equipment needed:

- paddle brush
- de-tangling comb
- styling comb
- tail comb
- hair grips/hairpins.

Prepare the hair first by setting or blow-drying as necessary, depending on the effect to be achieved.

1   Brush the hair thoroughly, starting from the ends and working up through the mid-lengths to the roots.

2   Brush or comb the hair to the centre left of the head, keeping the hair nice and flat.

3   Make sure the hair is smooth and held securely before placing the hair grips in a criss-cross position, overlapping each other up to the crown (a).

4   Place a grip in the opposite direction to stop the hair sliding out of the gripped area (b).

5   At this point back-combing can be added to the roots behind the gripped area. Handle the hair gently to avoid disrupting the hair grips. This will give support and create height to the finished French plait (c).

6   To create a smooth finish, comb the outer back section of the hair, apply oil sheen spray and holding spray and comb the hair again gently.

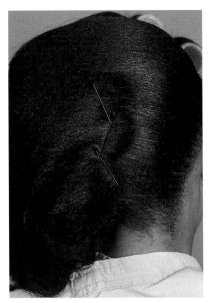

(a) Placing grips in a criss-cross pattern

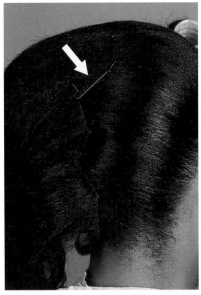

(b) Placing a grip in the opposite direction

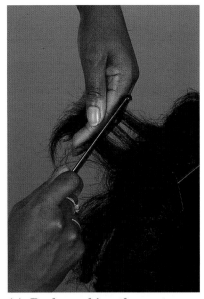

(c) Back-combing the roots

7 Hold the hair around the middle lengths and twist inwards, forming a coil (d). Secure the hair temporarily in this position with a large pin or section clip.

8 Smooth the outside of the pleat with a comb.

9 Smooth the surrounding hair, making sure all ends are secure. Apply oil sheen spray and then holding spray to the hair. Secure the French plait by using invisible pins bent at one end. This will ensure that the plait remains in place (e) & (f).

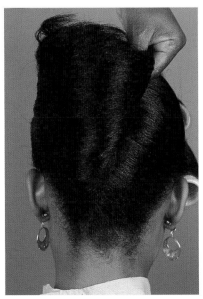

(d) Forming a coil

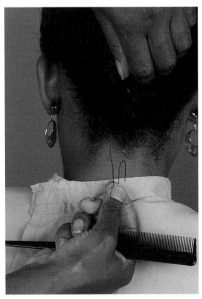

(e) A bent pin

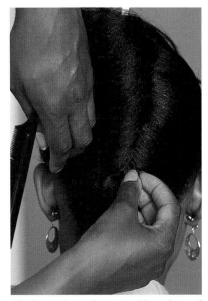

(f) Securing the outside edge of the plait with bent pins

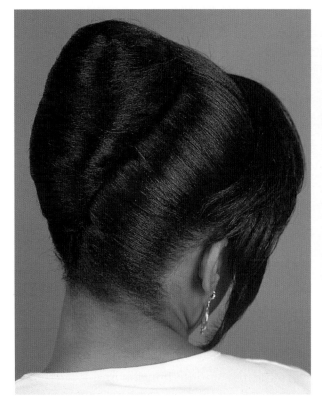

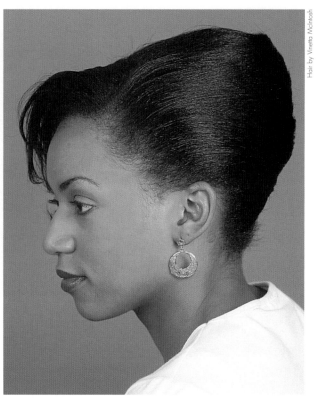

Hair by Vinetta McIntosh

The finished French plait

Desmond Murray

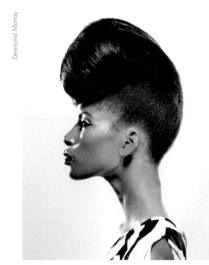

Horizontal roll

Tip

The wider the circle created, the wider the finished cluster will be.

Cluster of curls

This style is suitable for medium to long hair and is ideal for special occasions.

1   Wrap set or set the hair using the brick-setting technique. Comb the hair out and apply dressing or oil sheen spray to the hair. Blow-dry the hair and tong if necessary.

2   Part the hair on the side, leaving the fringe area out. Brush the hair on the sides and back upwards into a pony tail. Grip the hair in a circle and interlock the grips so that the hair is secure.

3   Take a section of hair and back-comb it. Smooth the top section of the hair (a).

4   Roll the hair into a curl and hold in place (b).

5   Fasten the formed curl with a grip or bent pin. Place curls on the outside around the perimeter near the grips first. This will build a foundation for the rest of the curls. Interlock the curls, building height in the crown (c).

6   Brush the fringe area into place. Spray the hair with oil sheen and holding spray.

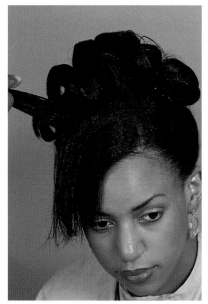

(a) Taking a section of hair

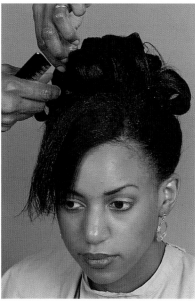

(b) Forming a curl

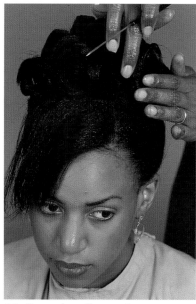

(c) Securing the curls

The finished style

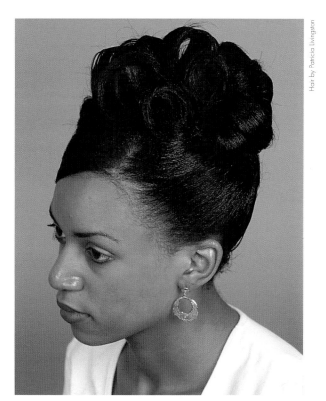

Hair by Patricia Livingston

Client aftercare

It is important that clients use the correct products to maintain the hairstyle between salon visits. The table lists aftercare products which are suitable for a variety of hairstyles. These products can be recommended to clients for use in between salon visits.

Hairstyle	Advice on aftercare	Finishing products
Shampoo and set; wrap set; blow-dry	Always use conditioner after shampooing the hair; conditioning treatment should be applied every 2 to 4 weeks depending on the condition of the hair and frequency of shampooing	Oil sheen spray; holding spray; hairdressing cream; serum.
Finger waves; push waves	Do not keep the hairstyle for longer than 2 weeks; the hairstyle should not be worn continually – other hair styling options should be used to avoid the scalp becoming too dry and hair breakage occurring	Regular use of oil sheen spray to give the hair sheen and moisturise the scalp; holding spray or spritz depending on the hold required.
Scrunch dry; permed hair	Shampoo and condition the hair every 1 to 2 weeks (very dry hair may require shampooing every 2 weeks) to allow the finishing products to penetrate the scalp and hair and the moisture balance to be built up; conditioning treatment should be applied every 2 to 3 weeks depending on the condition of the hair and frequency of shampooing	Activator and moisturiser; oil sheen spray to give shine; select the type of finishing product to be used depending on how dry the hair is and the effect to be created.

For further information see Chapter 3 and the section on finishing techniques in this chapter.

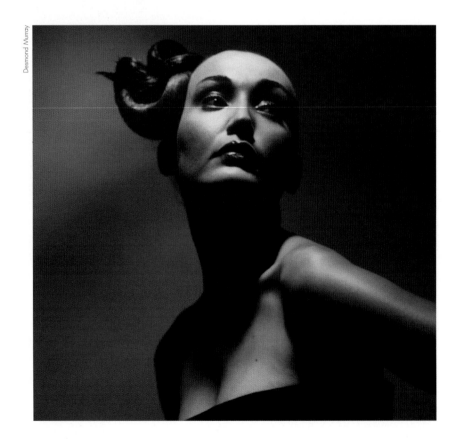

Desmond Murray

Chemical relaxing

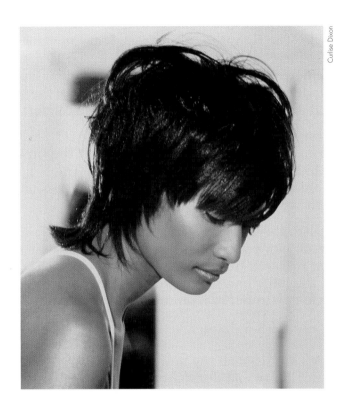

7

Curlise Dixon

Learning objectives

This chapter covers the following:

- **the science of relaxing**

- **consultation and analysis**

- **types of relaxer**

- **application of relaxer to virgin hair, regrowth and as a corrective measure**

Early hair straighteners used in the 1940s in America were made of a combination of lye, potato and eggs. This was a home made concoction, which would be prepared by the individual and applied to the hair. Vaseline would be used to protect the scalp. Nonetheless the product was extremely caustic, would burn the scalp and could damage the hair. This early formula was popular in the early 1940s and used in the main by young men who wanted to achieve a 'Konked' hairstyle. The Konk was an extremely fashionable hairstyle and the forerunner to the quiff worn in the 1950s. The look was achieved by straightening the hair and styling it with gel to produce a wavy/straight look, which was the height of fashion and obviously worth the initial discomfort.

Chemical relaxing, also known as straightening, first became popular in the 1960s. The products used at the time were not as sophisticated as present-day relaxers. The straightening products of the 1960s were not very successful, often resulting in very brittle hair and scalp damage.

The 1970s saw the rebirth of the straightener in a more sophisticated form, now called relaxer. Companies currently carry out a lot of research to ensure that their products are much kinder to the hair than previous ones. Today's relaxers are packed with buffers, protein and oil with the result that the hair retains more moisture and is left in a better condition.

Chemical relaxers are used on the hair to increase manageability, flexibility and durability when styling. The process involves relaxing or straightening the natural curl or wave in the hair. The chemical relaxing process is permanent – as the hair grows, the new growth will be naturally curly in contrast to the area that has been relaxed. The only way to remove relaxed hair is to let it grow out and cut it off, as once the hair is relaxed it will not revert back to its natural curl pattern.

Product development for chemical relaxers has been initiated by American companies. There has been increased research into the development of chemical relaxers in the UK and Europe, but America remains the leader in this type of research.

The science of relaxing

The hair is made up of keratin – a protein also found in nails and skin. Keratin gives the hair its tensile strength and elasticity, allowing the hair to be stretched. Each strand of hair is made up of three parts: **cuticle**, **cortex** and **medulla** (for further information on the structure of hair see Chapter 2).

Inside the hair

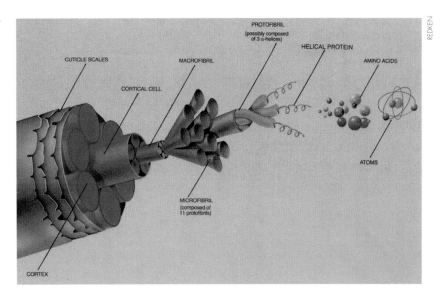

There are three bonds we are mainly concerned with when chemically processing, blow-drying, setting or thermally processing hair. These are **disulphide**, **salt** and **hydrogen** bonds. Disulphide or sulphur bonds are the strongest. These bonds are broken when the hair is relaxed or permed. If too many of these bonds are broken during the chemical process, the hair will become weak and break. Salt bonds and hydrogen bonds are weak and break when the hair is shampooed, blow-dried or set, reforming as the hair dries. Hydrogen bonds are broken when the hair is thermally processed.

If you look at an individual strand of African-Caribbean hair, some parts appear thicker than others. This uneven keratinisation causes the hair to become curly, with the cortex consisting of two types – **para cortex** and **ortho cortex** (for more information see Chapter 2).

When a chemical relaxer is applied to the hair, the product causes the cuticle to swell, allowing it to penetrate the cortex. The disulphide bonds in the cortex are broken and one sulphur atom is removed from the broken bond. They then rejoin with a new partner – **lanthionine**. The hair now has one sulphur bond and one lanthionine bond. Relaxed hair cannot be permed because in order for a perm to be effective the disulphide bond must be intact. After the relaxing process, one bond is permanently straight and cannot be altered.

Once the hair is relaxed sufficiently, the chemical relaxer is rinsed from the hair to halt the process. The hair is then shampooed using a neutralising shampoo which is acidic and removes any traces of alkaline which may still remain in the hair. The shampoo closes the cuticle and brings the hair back to its normal pH.

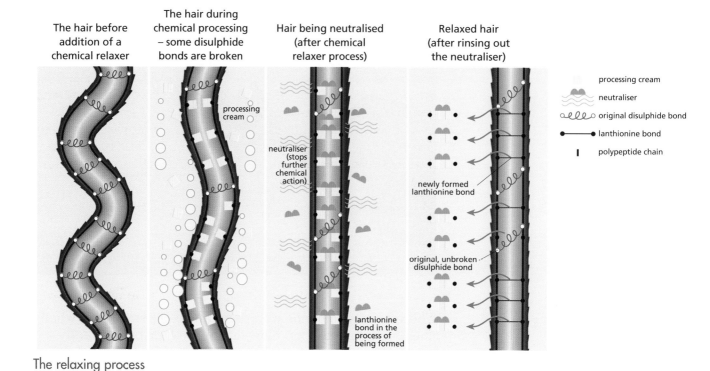

| The hair before addition of a chemical relaxer | The hair during chemical processing – some disulphide bonds are broken | Hair being neutralised (after chemical relaxer process) | Relaxed hair (after rinsing out the neutraliser) |

processing cream

neutraliser (stops further chemical action)

lanthionine bond in the process of being formed

newly formed lanthionine bond

original, unbroken disulphide bond

processing cream
neutraliser
original disulphide bond
lanthionine bond
polypeptide chain

The relaxing process

Relaxed hair should not be permed under any circumstances as this would result in the following:

● no curl pattern
● excessive damage and dryness, causing hair breakage.

In other words it would be a complete waste of time.

Consultation and analysis

Chemical relaxers can be applied in different situations:

● to virgin hair
● to regrowth on hair that has been relaxed previously
● to correct a previous uneven relaxing treatment.

Tip

Extreme caution must be used when applying a relaxer because the products used can cause irreparable damage.

These situations will be treated separately after a discussion of the safety precautions that need to be observed and the methods and techniques to be used when relaxing the hair. If the necessary care is taken during the consultation, analysis and application of any chemical process, this will minimise any damage to the scalp and hair.

Consultation prior to a relaxer treatment

An in-depth client consultation carried out prior to the application of any chemical process can avoid complications occurring during the application of products and after the chemical process has been completed. A properly structured consultation will help you construct your client history and prepare client records for present and future use. (For more information on consultation and analysis see Chapter 1.)

The consultation sheet on the next page lists questions that should be asked by a stylist when carrying out a consultation with the client prior to relaxing. The results of the consultation will provide you with the necessary information to enable you to decide whether or not the client's hair is suitable for relaxing. Record the information gained from the consultation on the record card.

The table lists conditions under which a relaxer should *not* be applied, together with corrective procedures.

Problem	Causes/effects	Solution
Psoriasis/ abrasions on the scalp	Psoriasis (for further information see Chapter 15); scratching the scalp prior to a chemical relaxer can cause abrasions on the scalp	Apply conditioning treatment to the scalp and hair; do not apply relaxer until the scalp has healed (A client experiencing a bad outbreak of psoriasis should seek medical advice). If the psoriasis is dormant and there are no abrasions a relaxer can be applied. As a precaution the scalp must be protected prior to processing.
Damaged, brittle hair	Too many chemical processes; overlapping of chemical relaxer; not enough conditioning treatments	Apply reconstructive conditioning treatment; cut off the over-processed hair; recommend a course of conditioning treatments.
Hair extensions	Removal of hair extensions 3–7 days prior to applying a relaxer could cause it to irritate the scalp	Apply a course of conditioning treatment to the hair (any hair that has just had extensions removed should have a course of conditioning treatment); relax hair after 2 weeks to 1 month provided hair is in good condition.
Hair has been shampooed within the last 3 days	Scalp could have become sensitised and cause the relaxer to irritate	Apply conditioning treatment; relax hair within 1 week once the hair is in a good condition.
Permanent colour/ bleach/highlights	Could cause the hair to become over-processed and brittle	Relax the hair 3 months after colouring; recommend a course of conditioning treatments.

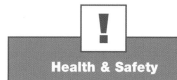

Health & Safety

On permanently coloured and bleached/highlighted hair, only relax the regrowth to avoid over-processing and hair breakage. Never relax hair that has been treated with metallic salts as this could cause the hair to break.

Tip

You can chemically relax hair where you have identified your client as having a naturally sensitive scalp by first applying a protective base (see later in this chapter).

CLIENT CONSULTATION SHEET

Client's name: Stylist's name:

Address: Date:

When did you last shampoo your hair?

When was your hair last relaxed?

Which product was used?

Were any problems experienced during the chemical relaxing process such as:

- scalp irritation
- insufficient processing
- hair breakage?

Have you recently had braids, extensions or hair weave removed from your hair?   yes / no

If yes, how long ago?

Have you had permanent colour on your hair?   yes / no

If yes, how long ago?

Has your hair been permed?   yes / no

If yes, how long ago?

When was your last conditioning treatment?

Do you know which product was used?   yes / no

If yes, please state name of conditioner.

Has your hair been thermally processed with a thermal comb or tong?   yes / no

If yes, how long ago?

Does your scalp ever become sensitive during the relaxing process?   yes / no

If yes, is it in isolated areas or the complete scalp?

Type of relaxer to be carried out: regrowth ☐ full head ☐ corrective ☐

Analysis

When analysing the scalp and hair before relaxing, you need to consider the following:

- condition of scalp and hair
- natural curl pattern (how curly or wavy the hair is)
- areas identified during the consultation process
- strength of product required
- processing time.

As part of your analysis you must carry out the following tests:

- elasticity test
- porosity test
- density test
- hair texture.

(Refer to Chapters 1 and 2 for further details of consultation, analysis and diagnostic tests.)

Elasticity test

If the hair is in a good condition, it will stretch and return to its normal length without breaking when you carry out this test. If the hair breaks, recommend a course of treatments to strengthen the hair. In extreme cases you may need to cut off the damaged hair. If breakage is not extreme, you can chemically relax the hair and then give a course of treatments afterwards.

Porosity test

If you find the hair to be extremely porous, recommend a course of conditioning treatment prior to relaxing. With normal or average porosity apply a pre-perm product to coat and protect the cuticle prior to relaxing. Avoid the relaxer coming into contact with previously processed hair. (Further information on pre-perm products is given later in this chapter.)

Scalp condition

Examine the scalp for abrasions and question the client on any sensitivity experienced during any previous relaxing processes. If abrasions are present, do not chemically process the hair.

Hair condition/natural curl pattern

Observe the natural curl pattern and hair texture, which will help you to establish the extent of the relaxation required and the correct strength of relaxer to use. Check the hair condition for signs of breakage. (For further information on natural curl pattern see Chapter 2.)

Hair texture

Assessing the clients' hair prior to chemically relaxing it is important, as it helps us to decide which strength product should be used.

Hair which has a thick texture may be resistant and require a super relaxer. Medium texture hair will need a regular relaxer, while fine texture hair requires a mild relaxer.

Scalp sensitivity

If your client has a sensitive scalp, you can protect the scalp by applying a protective base. Avoid using a heavy, oil-based scalp protector as excessive application could leave a barrier on the hair and prevent the relaxer from penetrating the cuticle, resulting in insufficient processing.

Relaxer strand test

This test is optional. If you are in any doubt about the strength of relaxer you need to use or whether your client's hair is in a good enough condition to be relaxed, you can carry out a pre-relaxer test by isolating and treating a small section of hair. The section taken should be in the nape area or where the hair is more resistant and should not be wider than 12 mm (half an inch).

- Use section clips to clip surrounding hair away.
- Cover clipped hair with a wad of cotton wool to prevent chemical relaxer from coming into contact with it.
- Apply the selected strength to the test section.
- Smooth and check strand every 3 minutes; observe the hair continuously.
- When the hair is relaxed sufficiently, rinse off the chemical thoroughly and apply neutralising shampoo.

If you decide to proceed with the relaxer on completion of the test, do not do this on the same day but apply a conditioning treatment to the hair. If the hair is in good condition you can apply the relaxer within 4–7 days. (Remember to omit the strand that has been previously tested when you carry out the chemical relaxer process.)

The results of the test will give you an indication of the following:

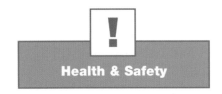

Health & Safety

Never apply relaxer to wet hair as this could cause breakage.

- whether the hair is in a good enough condition to be relaxed
- the strength of product to use
- the processing time
- the condition the hair would be in after the chemical relaxer has been applied.

Types of relaxer

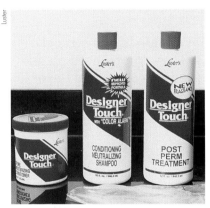

Relaxing products

There are five types of chemical relaxers:

- sodium hydroxide
- calcium hydroxide
- potassium hydroxide
- guanidine hydroxide
- lithium hydroxide.

All relaxers contain hydroxide. They all process the hair in the same way by opening the cuticle and penetrating the cortex where they break the disulphide bonds and cause the hair to become relaxed (straight). All relaxers are strongly alkaline, i.e. they have a high pH.

Product companies have divided relaxers into two types: **lye** and **no-lye** products. Sodium hydroxide relaxers are classified as lye products, while calcium, potassium, guanidine and lithium hydroxide relaxers are classified as no-lye.

Lye relaxers have a tendency to:

- be irritating to the scalp
- cause less drying of the hair
- leave the hair with more sheen
- penetrate the cuticle more quickly.

No-lye relaxers have a tendency to:

- be less irritating to the scalp
- be more drying on the hair and scalp – the hair will need to be moisturised more often to avoid dryness and breakage
- leave the hair in need of frequent conditioning treatments
- penetrate the cuticle more slowly.

There are exceptions: potassium hydroxide penetrates the cuticle rapidly and is not used that often in relaxers any more; guanidine hydroxide does not have as drying an effect on the hair as other no-lye relaxers; lithium hydroxide is less drying on the hair and produces a similar result to a sodium hydroxide relaxer but is kinder to the scalp.

Sodium hydroxide relaxers are available in three strengths, with a pH range of 12 to 13:

- **Super relaxer:** for resistant hair
- **Regular relaxer:** for normal hair
- **Mild relaxer:** for thin or colour-treated hair.

Calcium hydroxide relaxers are available in one strength only, with a pH range of 12 to 13. They can be used on all hair types. More recently, some product companies have produced a stronger 'resistant' strength for coarse, resistant hair.

Associated products

Pre-relaxer treatments

These are used on porous hair before application of the relaxer. They coat the cuticle with a polymer film which acts as a buffer to slow the action of the chemical product. They will not prevent the hair from becoming over-processed but by slowing down the process, they make it easier to control.

Tip

When working on clients with a sensitive scalp and providing no abrasions are present, use a protective base before applying a relaxer.

Protective base

A protective base is used to coat the scalp prior to applying a chemical relaxer. It usually has a petroleum base and is light to the touch, spreads easily on the scalp and is easily removed when the hair is shampooed after the relaxing process. It is usual to apply a protective base when working with sodium hydroxide relaxers. It is not usually necessary to use a protective base when using calcium hydroxide relaxers as these tend not to sensitise the scalp.

Tip

Not all product manufacturers produce a post-perm treatment. Some manufacturers produce a product that can be used across a range of relaxing products.

Post-perm treatments

A post-perm treatment is applied after the relaxer has been rinsed from the hair. These products are acidic and will bring the hair back to its normal pH level and moisturise the hair after the chemical relaxing process.

Neutralising shampoo

A neutralising shampoo is used after the hair has been relaxed sufficiently and all the product thoroughly rinsed out. It will cleanse the hair of any remaining relaxer and neutralise any alkalinity still present, bringing the hair back to its normal pH of around 5.5 and closing the cuticle.

Application of relaxer

Tip

It is important to take great care before and during application of a chemical relaxer. If your consultation and analysis have been thorough, you will avoid damage to the hair and scalp.

Tip

If in doubt as to whether the necessary degree of relaxation has been achieved, take a strand of hair and remove relaxer from it with a piece of cotton wool. You will then see whether the hair has been relaxed sufficiently.

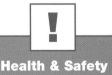

Health & Safety

If during the relaxing process there is any irritation to the scalp, rinse the relaxer off immediately and discontinue the process.

If the consultation, analysis and tests are positive you can now proceed with the chemical relaxer process. The following products and equipment are necessary before applying a chemical relaxer treatment:

- protective wear for client and self – towels, gown, plastic cape, rubber gloves
- protective base
- pre-relaxer treatment
- non-metallic tail comb, de-tangling comb, sectioning clips
- cotton wool
- relaxing product
- neutralising shampoo
- conditioner
- any other products recommended by the product company.

Procedure for chemical relaxer application to regrowth

1   Gown and protect your client with towels and plastic cape.
2   Apply a protective base to the skin just below the hairline, being careful not to apply protective base onto the hair as this could cause a barrier to the chemical relaxing treatment (a). If your client is sensitive to the relaxer apply protective base to the scalp also.
3   Apply a pre-relaxer treatment to the hair mid-lengths and ends of the hair which will not be chemically processed (b).
4   Divide the hair into four sections and protect your hands with rubber gloves. Dispense the product into a bowl.

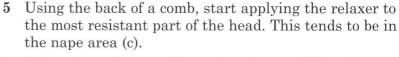

5 Using the back of a comb, start applying the relaxer to the most resistant part of the head. This tends to be in the nape area (c).

6 Take sub-sections no bigger than 6 mm (1/4 inch). Apply relaxer 6 mm away from the scalp.

It is necessary to apply the relaxer 6 mm away from the scalp because the chemical product expands after it is

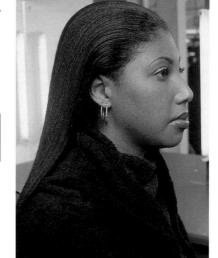

Before application

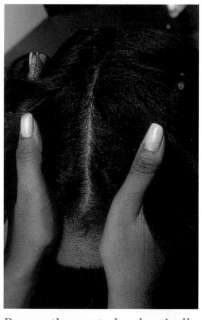

Regrowth area to be chemically relaxed

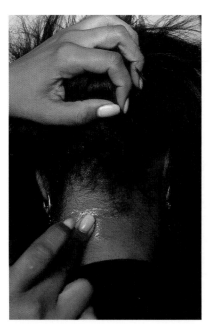

(a) Applying protector around the hairline

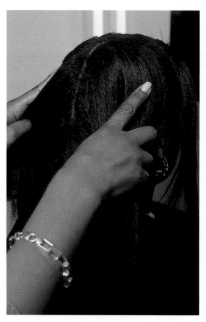

(b) Applying pre-relaxer to the mid lengths and ends

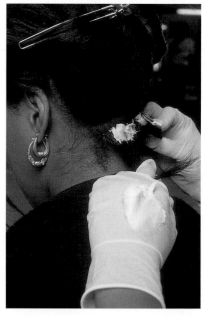

(c) Applying relaxer to the most resistant part of the hair, in the nape area

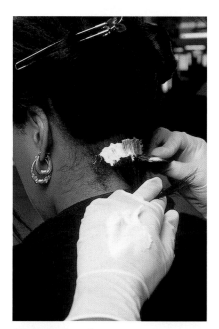

(d) Working from ear to ear

applied due to body temperature and the reaction of the hair to the chemical product. If the relaxer is applied too close to the scalp there will be no room for it to expand without coming into contact with the scalp, possibly causing irritation.

7   Apply the product to the hair working from ear to ear, rather than working on one quarter section of the head and then another (d).

The latter method could cause parts of the hair to be over-processed and other parts under-processed, resulting in an uneven finish. By using the former method of application you will ensure that the chemical relaxer result is methodical and consistent and you will achieve an even end result.

8   Hold the ends of the hair while you apply the relaxer so that the regrowth area can be clearly seen (e).

9   Continue to apply relaxer to the crown regrowth area, working up towards the front of the hairline. Just lay the product onto the hair – make sure you do not comb the relaxer into the rest of the hair at this stage as this could damage the hair (f) & (g).

10 Once you have applied relaxer to the whole of the regrowth area, go back to the area where you first started your application. Start by combing the regrowth area only and smoothing it with your fingers (h), (i), (j), (k) & (l).

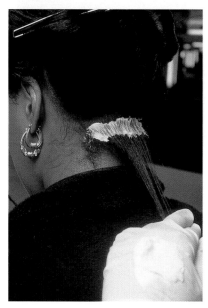

(e) Holding ends of the hair so that regrowth area can be seen clearly

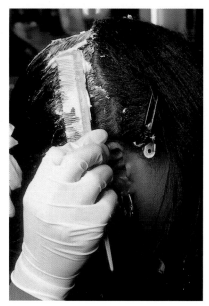

(f) Applying relaxer to the crown regrowth area

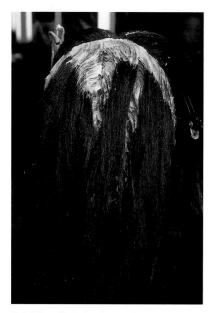

(g) The finished application

Tip

Hold the hair gently; do not pull the hair as this could cause the scalp to become irritated.

Health & Safety

Do not flood the hair with too much relaxer as this could cause over-processing.

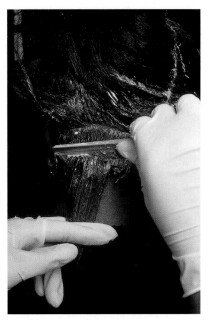

(h) Starting the relaxing process by gently combing the regrowth area

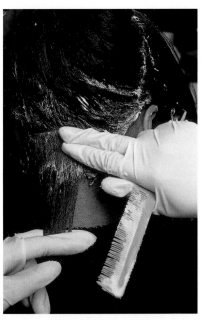

(i) Smoothing the section after combing

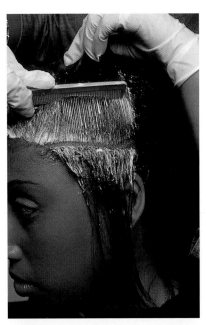

(j) Combing and smoothing the sides

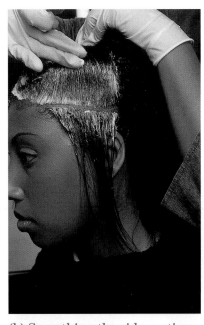

(k) Smoothing the side section after combing

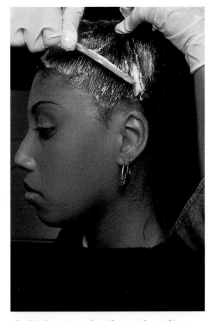

(l) Relaxing the front hairline

Health & Safety

Never relax the hair 100 per cent as the hair will become too straight and liable to break.

Do not comb beyond the regrowth area as this could cause overlapping. Take care not to scrape the scalp as you work with the hair as this could sensitise the scalp. It is kinder to the hair and less damaging to use your fingers to smooth the hair. Do not be tempted to use the back of the comb to smooth the hair as this is a harder object and could cause hair breakage and sensitise the scalp.

Tip

Hair can be relaxed to remove some of the natural curl. This technique is called texturising and is ideal on short hairstyles or styles that require minimum straightening.

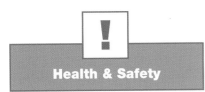

Health & Safety

Always follow manufacturer's recommendations on application and removal procedures.

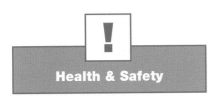

Health & Safety

Never use hot water to rinse the hair as this could cause scalp irritation and burn the scalp. If the scalp has become sensitive during the relaxing process, rinse with cold water.

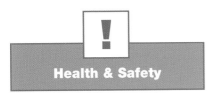

Health & Safety

Do not massage or rub the scalp vigorously as this could cause it to become irritated and sensitised.

As you work the relaxer through the hair, apply more product to those areas where coverage is not sufficient and even. You will be doing two things at this stage – cross checking your application and continuing to chemically relax the hair. Using this method of application will mean that you can work through the hair more quickly and efficiently. It will result in a more accurate application and at the same time be more effective.

Once you have worked completely through the hair, if the hair still needs to be straighter start processing the hair again from the area where you first started your application, combing and smoothing the relaxer only up to the regrowth area. Once this has been completed the hair should now be relaxed. To check if the hair is relaxed sufficiently, take a strand of hair and remove the relaxer with cotton wool. Once the hair does not revert to its original curl and keeps the newly formed relaxed formation, the product can be removed.

Rinsing

11 If the hair is relaxed sufficiently, start rinsing the hair thoroughly, using tepid water. Allow the force of the water spray to flush the chemical relaxer out from roots to points. While rinsing, use your fingers gently to assist removal of the relaxer from the scalp and hair; this will help to prevent the scalp being sensitised (m).

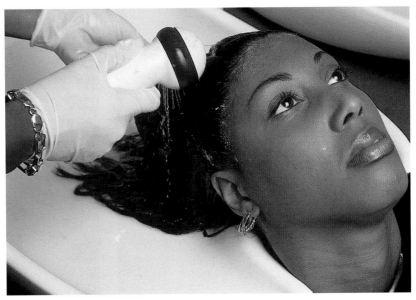

(m) Rinsing the relaxer off

Tip

For hair that is in poor condition it is better to set the hair after relaxing rather than blow-drying as this can put undue stress on the hair.

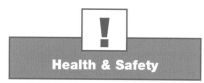

Health & Safety

Relaxer left in the hair can cause the hair to break and damage the scalp.

12 Once you have finished rinsing, check to make sure all traces of the relaxing chemical have been removed from the scalp and hair and apply post-perm treatment.

Neutralising

13 Apply a neutralising shampoo to the hair. Shampoo gently but thoroughly, taking care to make sure all areas of the scalp are massaged. Rinse thoroughly.

14 Re-apply shampoo and rinse thoroughly. The hair should be shampooed at least twice to ensure that all the chemical relaxer has been removed. It is important that you rinse the hair thoroughly after shampooing.

15 Towel-dry the hair.

16 Comb the hair to ensure it is tangle free. Apply styling lotion of your choice.

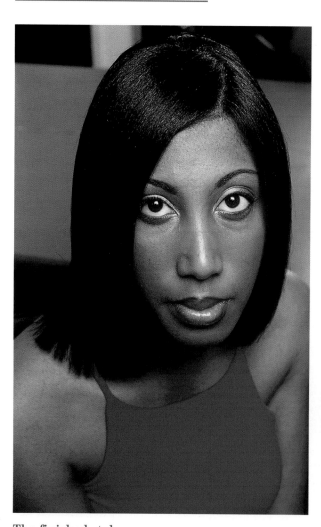
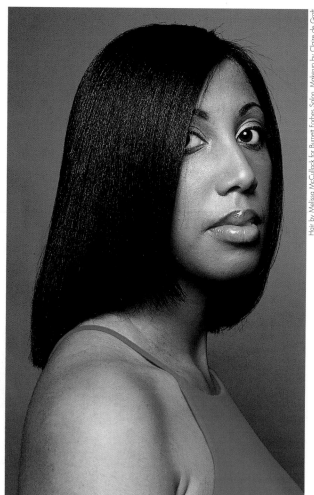

Hair by Melissa McCullock for Burnett Forbes Salon. Makeup by Claire de Graft

The finished style

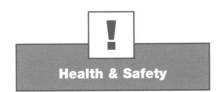

If the scalp is sensitive apply a protective base, take care not to over-saturate the hair as it could act as a barrier.

17 Style as desired.

18 Fill in a record card.

Procedure for chemical relaxer application to virgin hair

Complete all the tests as described in regrowth relaxer application. Select your products and equipment as before.

1 Apply pre-relaxer treatment if the hair is dry and slightly porous. If the hair is in good condition, there is no need to apply any pre-relaxer treatment.

2 Apply a protective base around the hairline.

3 Divide the hair into four sections.

4 Apply relaxer to the mid-lengths and ends first. Starting from the most resistant part of the head or nape area, work upwards towards the crown and forward towards the front hairline.

5 Once you have applied relaxer to mid-length and ends throughout the head, start applying relaxer to the root area, taking care to apply relaxer 6 mm away from the scalp. Work from the nape area up to the front hairline as before.

6 Start combing and smoothing the hair with the fingers, taking 6 mm (0.25 inch) sub-sections of hair. Work from ear to ear, applying more relaxer where necessary. Once this has been completed, comb through the hair from roots to ends and smooth with the fingers. Work with the hair until the required degree of relaxing is achieved as in regrowth relaxer application.

7 Rinse the hair thoroughly, following steps 11–14 as in regrowth relaxer application. Style as desired.

8 Fill in a record card.

Applying a corrective chemical relaxer treatment

A corrective chemical relaxer will need to be applied to any head of hair where the relaxing process is uneven. The table illustrates some problems that can occur during chemical relaxing and procedures that can be used to correct them.

Problem	Causes/effects	Solution
Ends of the hair under-processed	Relaxer not left on the ends of the hair for long enough. Calcium hydroxide relaxer used on the ends, sodium hydroxide relaxer used on the roots	Apply relaxer to the ends and process until the desired result is achieved. Do not apply sodium hydroxide relaxer to the ends, as the hair will not become straighter and more damage will be caused; treat the hair on a regular basis with a reconstructive conditioner; cut regularly.
Mid-section of the hair is under-processed; roots and ends processed evenly	Relaxer has not been left on for long enough in this section; incorrect strength of relaxer used	Apply relaxer to mid-section and process until evenly matched with the roots and ends of the hair. **Do not** process if calcium hydroxide relaxer has been used previously.
Roots of the hair under-processed; ends straight	Relaxer has not been left on the roots for long enough; incorrect strength relaxer used	Apply relaxer to the root area only; process until evenly matched.

Tip

Sodium hydroxide and calcium hydroxide relaxers are not compatible. Once the hair has been processed with a calcium hydroxide relaxer, if it is not straight enough you should not try to relax the hair with sodium hydroxide relaxer, as it will not have any effect.

Tip

Corrective relaxing technique can be carried out to avoid hair breakage. Unevenly processed hair becomes weakened and will break easily during combing.

CASE STUDY

Karen's hair is shoulder length, normal texture and medium density. The hair was relaxed three months ago with a sodium hydroxide relaxer and the natural hair (regrowth area to be relaxed) has a medium curl pattern. There is no artificial colour on the hair. The ends of the hair are dry and will need cutting. Prior to the last chemical relaxer, Karen had not had a relaxer for five months. When the hair was relaxed the product was not left on long enough and the hair was under-processed. To avoid hair breakage and the under-processed mid-lengths becoming frizzy when styling, the hair must be relaxed again. A chemical relaxer will be applied to the regrowth area first and then combed through to the mid-length of the hair only to correct under-processed ends.

The following corrective chemical relaxer application relates to the case study above.

Step-by-step corrective chemical relaxer application

1 Carry out diagnostic tests for elasticity, porosity and density as previously described.
2 Apply protector around the front hairline and pre-protector to mid-lengths and ends.
3 Start application at the nape area (the most resistant part of the head on this client) (a).
4 Lay the relaxer on with a comb (b).

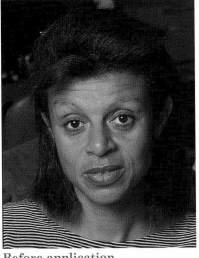

Before application

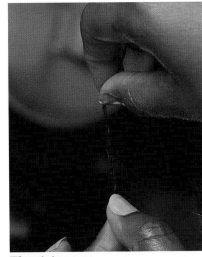

Elasticity test

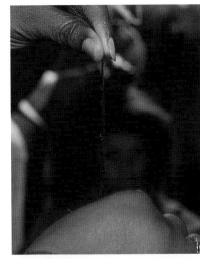

Porosity test

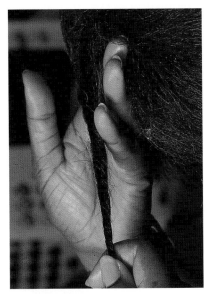

Density test

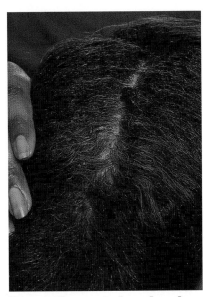

Regrowth area to be relaxed

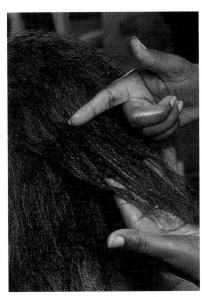

Mid-length area where the chemical corrective relaxer will be applied

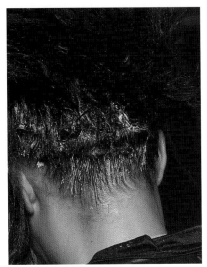

(a) Applying relaxer to the regrowth area

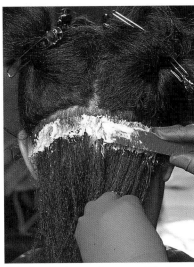

(b) Applying relaxer with the back of a comb

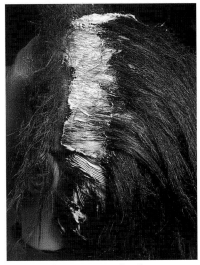

(c) Working towards the crown

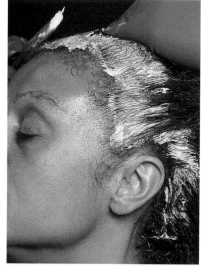

(d) Applying relaxer to the front hairline

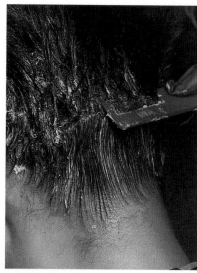

(e) Combing regrowth in the nape area

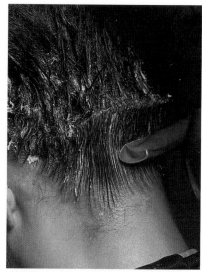

(f) Smoothing regrowth with the fingers

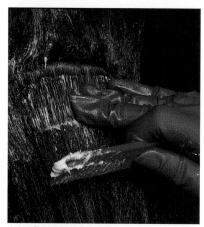

(g) Continuing the processing

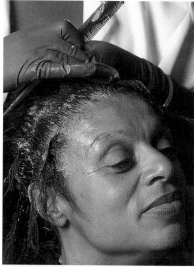

(h) Combing and smoothing the front hairline

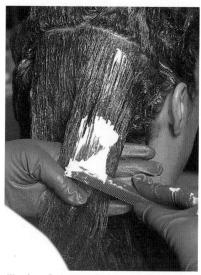

(i) Applying relaxer to the mid-lengths

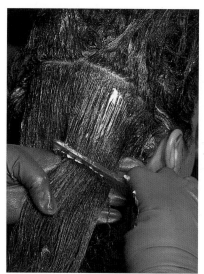

(j) Combing the mid-lengths

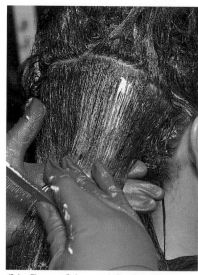

(k) Smoothing with the fingers

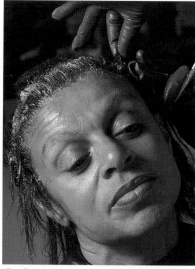

(l) Smoothing the front hairline

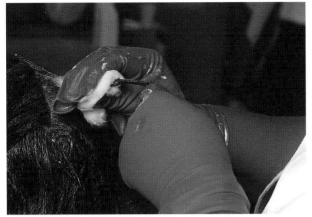

(m) Removing relaxer from a strand to ensure sufficient processing

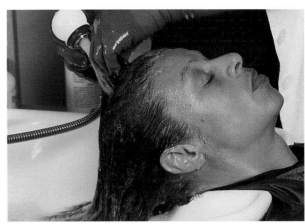

(n) Rinsing relaxer from the hair

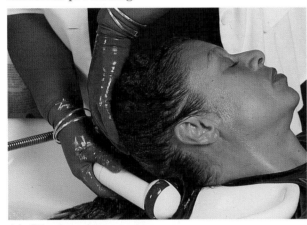

(o) Rinsing the nape area

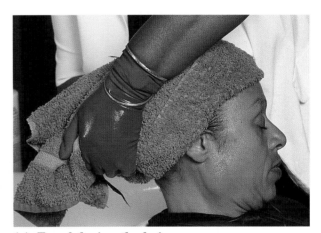

(p) Towel-drying the hair

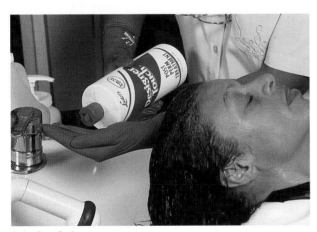

(q) Applying post-perm treatment

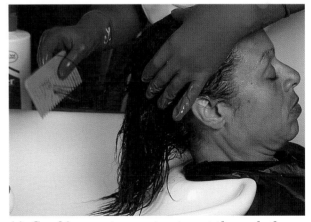

(r) Combing post-perm treatment through the hair

5 Work up the head towards the crown (c).

6 Apply relaxer to the front hairline (d).

7 Go back to the nape area and start combing and smoothing with the fingers (e) & (f).

8 Continue processing the hair using the same technique until you get to the front hairline (g) & (h).

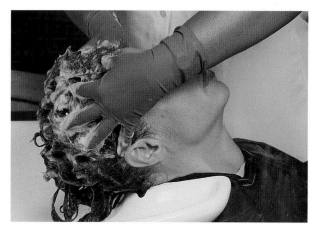

(s) Applying neutralising shampoo

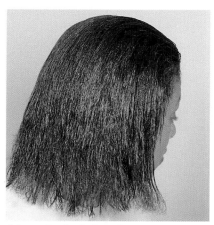

After the hair has been neutralised

The finished result after setting and styling

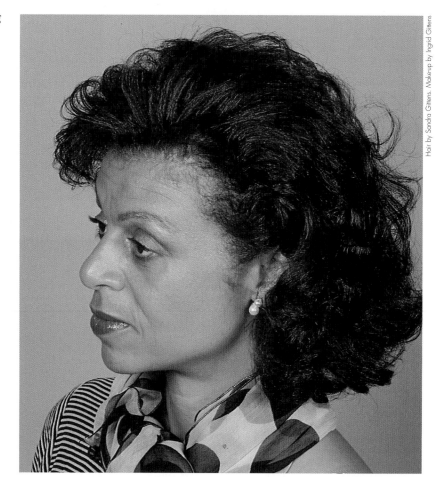

Hair by Sandra Gittens. Make-up by Ingrid Gittens

9   Go back to the nape area and apply more relaxer to the under-processed mid-length area (i).

10   Comb the hair from the regrowth to the mid-length (j).

11   Smooth the hair with the fingers (k).

12   Continue the process until you reach the front hairline (l).

Tip

When rinsing the hair, do not rub the scalp as there may still be relaxer present which could cause the scalp to become irritated. Lift the hair when rinsing chemical relaxer and allow the power of the water to remove the product.

13 Remove relaxer from a small strand of hair with a piece of cotton wool to ensure the hair is sufficiently relaxed (m).

14 Rinse the chemical relaxer thoroughly from the hair, making sure all product is removed from the nape area (n) & (o).

15 Towel dry the hair (p).

16 Apply post-perm treatment if recommended by the product company. Comb post-perm treatment through the hair (q) & (r). (Follow the manufacturer's instructions on the use of the post-perm treatment.)

17 Apply neutralising shampoo. Shampoo the hair twice to ensure all chemical relaxer is removed. Rinse the hair thoroughly (s).

18 Towel dry the hair; apply styling lotion and style as desired.

19 Fill in a record card.

Perming

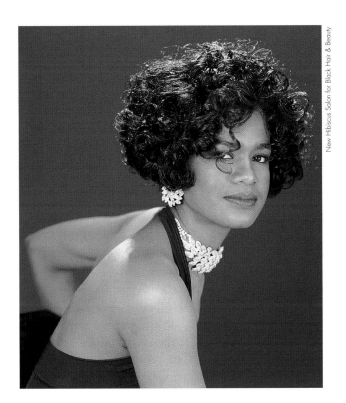

New Hibiscus Salon for Black Hair & Beauty

8

Learning objectives

This chapter covers the following:

- **the science of perming**
- **consultation and analysis**
- **product selection**
- **perm winding techniques**
- **regrowth perm application**
- **virgin hair application**

Perming African-Caribbean hair is a technique that was created in the mid 1970s. The process was developed by Jheri Redding, who devised the concept of perming African-Caribbean hair. The early perms were called a 'Jehri Curl' after its inventor. Perms went on to be called a wet look or Californian curl, because of the finishing products used at the time, which gave definition to the curl and produced a highly glossed, oily finish to the permed hair. As this look became unfashionable the term 'curly perm' was used.

This look is now commonly described and understood within the African-Caribbean industry as a '**perm**'.

Permanent waving is a term used to describe all types of waving systems which create an artificial curl or wave in the hair which remains there permanently until it is cut off, or grows out. If the hair is not cut the perm will grow further away from the scalp until eventually the hair reaches the end of its growing period and falls out.

When perming African-Caribbean hair, we are rearranging the curl pattern of the naturally curled hair so that we get a larger curl diameter and a more structured curl pattern. This allows the client to have greater manageability and freedom of style. It is important to remember that among African-Caribbean people, there are over 40 different hair types. When we refer to hair types, we are looking at the variety of curl patterns, which can vary from tight curly to wavy in texture. It is also not uncommon to find more than one curl pattern on one head, for example tighter curls towards the nape of the head and a looser curl pattern towards the crown or vice versa. Because of the variety of curl pattern which may be found on a single head of hair, a thorough consultation and analysis is important before perming the hair.

Tip

The pH of perms used on African-Caribbean hair is 9.5 and above.

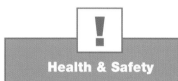

Health & Safety

Care must be taken when working with hair that has perm product on it. The hair is now in a fragile state as the disulphide bonds have been broken and these are fundamental to the strength of the hair. Irreparable damage can occur at this stage if the hair is handled roughly.

The science of perming

There are two types of perms used on African-Caribbean hair:

- one step perms or single action perms
- two step perms or dual action perms.

The active chemical found in most perms is **ammonium thioglycollate**. However, most perms used on African-Caribbean hair are dual action perms, sometimes called two step perms. These products tend to be kinder to the hair.

- The **single action perm** remains on the hair throughout the chemical process, first to smooth and

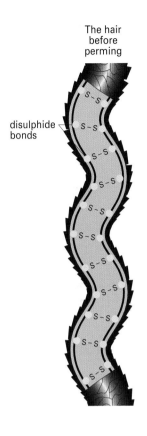

The hair before perming

disulphide bonds

straighten the hair. The hair is then wound onto the rods and the desired curl pattern is produced.

- In **dual action perms**, the first application of ammonium thioglycollate is usually in the form of a cream. This is step one and is called a 'rearranger'. The first step straightens and smoothes the hair in preparation for winding. The second step is the winding stage and the hair is wound with a weaker solution of ammonium thioglycollate which produces the curl pattern in the hair.

By a chemical process known as 'reduction' the hair structure is gradually softened, allowing it to straighten out the hair's natural curl. To do this the ammonium thioglycollate breaks many of the disulphide bonds in the hair, donating hydrogen atoms to prevent them reforming.

The concentrated cream rearranger is then thoroughly rinsed from the hair. The hair in its now pre-softened state is wound onto the **perming rods** or **rollers**. Prior to winding, a second application of ammonium thioglycollate, in the form of the winding lotion, is used. This is a weaker lotion and therefore less damaging to the hair. Disulphide bonds continue to be broken while the hair takes on its new shape which is dictated by the diameter of the rods or rollers.

Once the hair has been processed with the rods or curlers in place, it is then rinsed thoroughly. **Neutraliser** is then applied

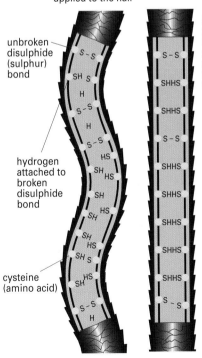

The disulphide bonds of the hair are broken when rearranger is applied to the hair

unbroken disulphide (sulphur) bond

hydrogen attached to broken disulphide bond

cysteine (amino acid)

Hair after the rearranger has been applied is now straighter and more flexible for winding

the sulphur atoms don't always line up with their partners

Reduction

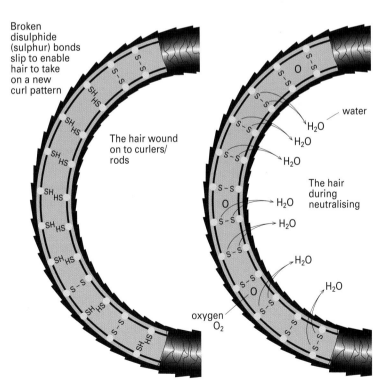

Broken disulphide (sulphur) bonds slip to enable hair to take on a new curl pattern

The hair wound on to curlers/ rods

oxygen O_2

water

The hair during neutralising

Winding before oxidation   Neutralising causes oxidation to the hair. The chemical action of the neutraliser is 'oxidation', which is the chemical opposite of reduction. Oxygen provided by the neutraliser removes the hydrogen from the broken disulphide bonds. The disulphide bonds can then reform in new positions to fix the hair into its new curl. Within the hair, cysteine once again becomes cystine.

Consultation

Consultation prior to a permanent wave is a very important part of any hairdressing service. Correct consultation and analysis will avoid long-term damage to the hair after a chemical process.

The following consultation sheet contains questions you should ask your client prior to perming the hair. This

PERMANENT WAVING CONSULTATION SHEET

Client's name: Stylist's name:

Address: Date:

When was your hair last permed?

Which product was used?

Were there any problems during or after your last perm?   yes/no
(e.g. scalp irritation, hair breakage/hair loss, other)

When did you last shampoo your hair?

When was your last conditioning treatment?

Do you know which product was used?   yes/no

If yes, please state name of product.

Have you recently had braids, extensions, hair weave
removed from your hair?   yes/no
If yes, how long ago?

Have you had permanent colour/bleach on your hair?   yes/no
If yes how long ago?

Has your hair been relaxed?   yes/no
If yes, how long ago?

Have you experienced any hair breakage?   yes/no

Has your hair been thermally processed with a thermal
comb or tong?   yes/no
If yes, how long ago?

Does your scalp ever become sensitive during the
perming process?   yes/no
If yes, is it in isolated areas or the complete scalp?

State type of perm to be carried out   regrowth   ☐

                                        full head   ☐

information, coupled with your analysis will tell you the condition of your client's hair and whether or not the hair can be chemically processed.

The client's answers to the above will help you decide whether or not you should proceed with a chemical process.

The following contra indication table outlines when a perm should or should not be given by listing problems you may come across when perming, and suitable action to be taken to solve the problems.

Problem	Course of action	Solution
Braids, extension, hair weave removed within the last week	Do not perm	Give a course of conditioning treatment if the hair is in a good condition – perm after 2 weeks to 1 month; hair in poor condition will need a prolonged course of conditioning treatments.
Hair thermally processed within the last week	Do not perm	Give a course of conditioning treatments; perm hair after 4 weeks to 2 months, providing no thermal processing remains in the hair and the hair is in a good condition.
Hair permanently coloured/ bleached within the last month	Do not perm	Give a course of conditioning treatments; perm within 2 to 3 months of permanent colour providing the hair is in a good condition; keep perm to regrowth only; protect ends; do not process colour-treated ends.
Hair breaking and weak	Do not perm	Give a course of conditioning treatment; cut damaged hair if necessary to avoid further breakage; do not perm until hair condition improves.
Hair permanently coloured 2 to 3 months ago	A perm can be carried out (once the hair is in a good condition)	Protect the ends; keep perm product on the regrowth only.
Hair previously relaxed	Do not perm (see Chapter 7)	Give regular conditioning treatments; the hair should not be permed until there is at least 6 months regrowth; all previously relaxed hair must be cut off.

Analysis

When analysing the scalp and hair prior to perming, you need to consider the following factors:

- condition of scalp and hair
- natural curl pattern (how curly or wavy the hair is)
- areas identified during the consultation process
- strength of product required
- processing time.

As part of your analysis you must carry out the following tests.

- porosity test
- elasticity test
- hair texture test (thick, normal, fine)
- perm test (depending on the condition of the hair).

Discuss with your client the type of curl/style required. If all the above tests are positive, you can carry out a perm. (Please refer to Chapter 1 in order to carry out the above tests correctly.)

Product selection

Tip

When carrying out a perm test, do not place rods too near the front hairline as this is the more sensitive area of the head and will process more quickly.

The responses to the questions asked during the consultation should tell you whether or not the client's hair may safely be permed and which product should be selected.

If there is any doubt regarding either of the above, a perm test should be carried out. This test will also help if you are not sure whether the hair is strong enough to be permed or which strength of product to use. It will also help you decide which size of rod or roller to use, and give an indication of processing time and curl result. Please use the contra indication table on the previous page as a guide when making your decision on whether or not to carry out a perm test.

Perm test

You will need the following items and products in order to complete a perm test:

- tint brush
- tail comb

Tip

If in doubt of the strength of rearranger to use, you could carry out your perm test with two different strengths of perm, e.g. super, regular or regular mild, depending on the strength of the hair and natural curl pattern.

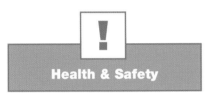

Health & Safety

Keep the application of different strength rearrangers on separate rods.

Tip

The time spent in carrying out a perm test will ensure the best end results with the minimum damage to the hair, meaning a happier client.

Tip

Not every company produces extra super strength perms.

- perm rod or curlers
- rearranger.

Procedure

- Do not pre-shampoo the hair.
- Select the size of rod or curler you intend to use.
- Take sections of hair the width and depth of a perm rod.
- Place one rod at the nape, one at the crown and one at the side of the head.

If you intend to carry out a regrowth application when perming your client's hair, apply cream rearranger to the regrowth area only. If it is a virgin application apply the rearranger to the whole length of the hair.

Wind the hair on the selected rod/roller. Leave the hair to process for 5–10 minutes only. Test the 'S' curl (shape developed). This will give you an indication of the following:

- which strength of rearranger to use
- which size rods or rollers to use
- the finished result that will be achieved
- the processing time
- the condition the hair will be left in after perming.

Types of perm

Perms come in three or four different strengths:

- extra super/maximum
- super
- regular
- mild.

Two main types of perm are used on African-Caribbean hair – **curly perm** and **body perm** or **body wave**. Both produce quite different end results:

- A curly perm produces a tighter, firmer look with solid curls. This perm is used on clients who prefer a more traditional 'permed' style in which the curls form the basis of the hairstyle.
- A body perm or body wave produces a softer, freer look and is for the client who enjoys the flexibility of wearing her hair in a soft curl or wave. Hair with a

body perm can also be set to produce a straighter look.

Pre-perm treatments

A pre-perm treatment should be used on hair which is porous from previous perm treatments. Pre-perm treatments coat the hair with a protective polymer film. This evens out the porosity of the cuticle and acts as a buffer against the chemical action of the perm product. Pre-perm treatments slow down the action of the chemical product but can not prevent the hair from becoming over-processed.

Perm winding techniques

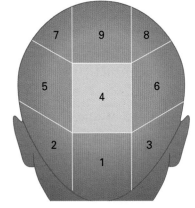

Nine section method

A variety of perm winding techniques can be used on African-Caribbean hair:

- nine section winding
- brick winding
- directional winding
- spiral winding.

Nine section winding

This is a methodical system of winding. The hair is divided into nine sections which allows the hair to be wound neatly within each section. The nine section technique is ideal for students who are beginning hairdressing (see illustration).

Brick winding

This technique is ideal for African-Caribbean hair. It allows the perm rods or rollers to sit closer to each other and avoids gaps and demarcation lines developing in the finished style. The hair is wound by placing rods or rollers in a brick pattern, similar to tiles on a roof (see illustration on page 50).

Directional winding

This technique is used to wind the hair in the direction it is to be styled after perming. For example, if the hair is worn with a side parting, establish the parting and then wind the hair to the side. If the hair is styled away from the face, wind the rods/rollers away from the face.

Winding the hair directionally will increase the durability of the finished hairstyle.

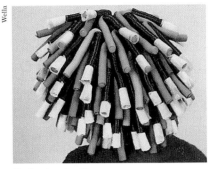

Spiral winding

Spiral winding

This technique is used to produce spiral curls on hair which is shoulder length and longer. The hair is wound by taking vertical sections and winding the hair from ends to roots. The hair is divided into nine sections prior to spiral winding to allow all sections to be wound neatly. The brick winding technique can also be used when spiral winding.

Rod/Roller size

The size of the rod or roller selected is dependent on several things:

- the type of curl desired
- the length of the hair
- the style in which the hair has been cut
- client requirements.

The larger the curl or rod selected, the softer and looser the end result will be; the smaller the rod or roller the tighter the end result. Variety, texture and support can be achieved by winding the hair with alternate large and small rods or rollers. This will produce a soft look with more texture and support in the finished style.

General winding techniques

When winding the hair, it is important to avoid fish-hook ends developing by ensuring the tips of the hair are wound smoothly around the rod or roller. A fish-hook end will produce a bent end on completion of the perm which will have to be cut off.

Perm rod or roller placement

The following points should be observed when winding the hair:

- The section taken must be no wider or deeper than the perm rod or roller. This will allow the rod or

Tip

When securing rollers with plastic pins, make sure that the pin is passed through the side of the roller where there is no hair and not through the middle of the roller, which could cause irreparable damage as the hair has got a chemical solution on it.

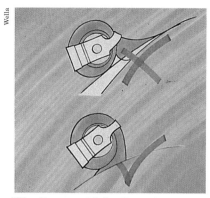

Winding – width of section

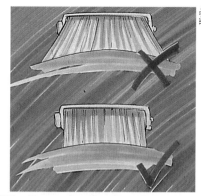

Winding – depth of section

Winding

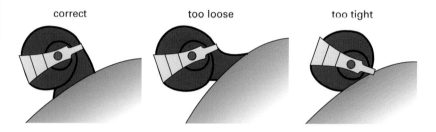

correct   too loose   too tight

roller to sit on its own base and avoid root drag and straight roots in the finished perm.

- The section taken when perm winding long hair must be slightly narrower than the perm rod or roller to avoid the hair spreading over the edges.

- Avoid fracture marks by making sure rubber bands on the perm rods are not placed too close to the hairline, as this could cause the hair to break at this point.

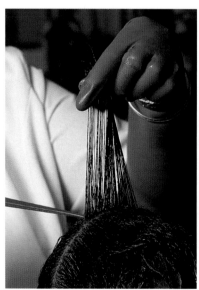

Sectioning

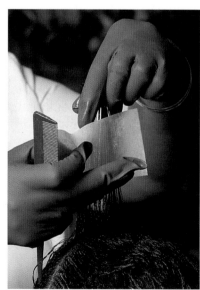

Application of end paper

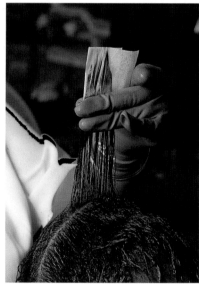

End paper folded in over the ends of the hair

Tip

Always follow manufacturer's instructions and health and safety recommendations. Never mix products from different perming systems – always keep to products recommended in the perming system you have selected to ensure best results.

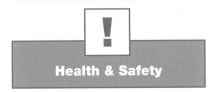

Health & Safety

If any irritation develops during the perm process, rinse off the chemical product immediately.

- Make sure the hair is combed smoothly and the end papers are placed on the ends of the hair and held securely to avoid frizzy ends in the finished perm. The illustrations on the previous page show the correct sectioning of the hair and application of end papers prior to winding the hair on rods or rollers.

The following products and equipment are necessary for applying a perm treatment:

- protective wear for client and self, towels, gowns, plastic cape, plastic tabbard, rubber gloves
- non-metal tail comb, de-tangling comb
- tinting brush
- perm rods/rollers
- shampoo as recommended by the manufacturer
- protective base
- pre-perm product
- selected perm products
- conditioner
- plastic cap
- end papers.

Regrowth perm application

Tip

You may not need to put a plastic cap on fine hair as it does not normally require additional heat.

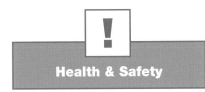

Health & Safety

Follow manufacturer's timings as these will vary according to the product. Do not leave the hair too long without checking as it could easily become over-processed.

1   Gown your client; protect your client with towels and a plastic cape.
2   Check the condition of the scalp and carry out elasticity, porosity and density tests.
3   Shampoo the hair gently once, using the shampoo recommended by the manufacturer (a).
4   Apply protective base to the skin just below the hairline, being careful not to get it onto the hair as this could create a barrier to the perming process (b).
5   Apply pre-perm treatment to the hair which isn't to be chemically processed (c).
6   Protect your hands with rubber gloves.
7   Divide the hair into four sections (d).
8   Using a tinting brush, start by applying rearranger to the most resistant part of the hair. This is usually at the back of the head between the ears and nape area (e).
9   Take sub-sections no bigger than 6 mm (0.25 inches) from ear to ear and apply rearranger 6 mm away from the scalp to allow for expansion. It is better to apply

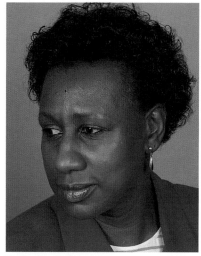

Before application

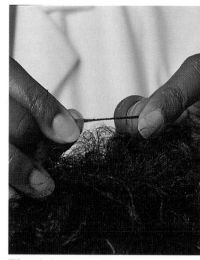

Elasticity test

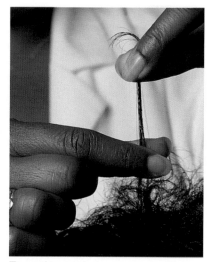

Porosity test

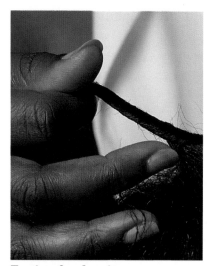

Testing for density

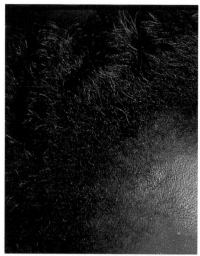

Regrowth area to be permed – front hairline

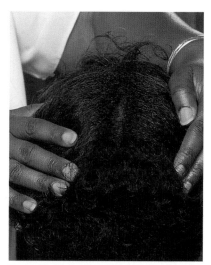

Regrowth area to be permed

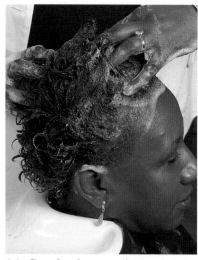

(a) Gentle shampooing prior to perming

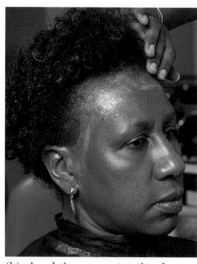

(b) Applying a protective base

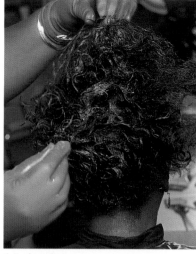

(c) Applying pre-perm treatment

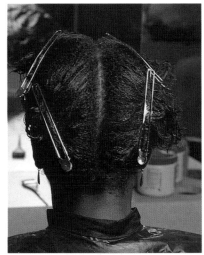

(d) The hair sectioned into four

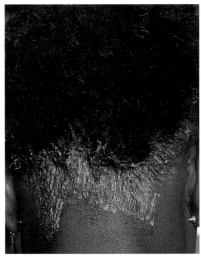

(e) Applying rearranger to the nape area

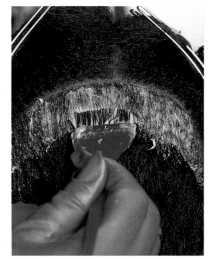

(f) Applying the product throughout the head

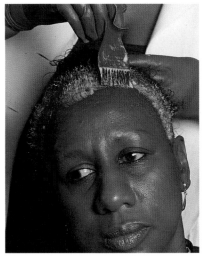

(g) Applying the product to the front hairline

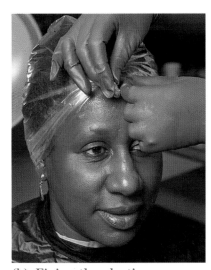

(h) Fixing the plastic cap

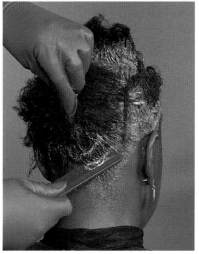

(i) Combing the regrowth area

Tip

The size of rods/rollers will determine how tight or loose the curls will be. A combination of smaller and larger rollers/rods alternately throughout the head will ensure a firm but soft shape.

the product to sections of the hair working from ear to ear, rather than working on one quarter section of the head at a time, as otherwise the quarter section treated first will have product on it for longer than the other sections. The last section treated could be under-processed as the product may not be left on for long enough. This could lead to an unevenly processed head of hair. Working from ear to ear will ensure that the perm process is methodical and consistent (f) & (g).

10   Once you have applied rearranger to all of the hair, cross check the application to make sure that the whole head is evenly covered with product.

11   Put on a plastic cap and allow the hair to process (h). If the salon is cold, wrap a towel around the head to give additional warmth.

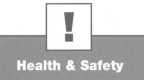

Health & Safety

Make sure all product is rinsed from the hair as perm left in the hair could cause irreparable damage to scalp and hair.

12   Process the hair for 10–20 minutes, check to see how the hair is processing every 10 minutes. Once the hair shows signs of the natural curl becoming straight, start combing the hair (i).

13   Comb the hair gently at the regrowth only and smooth with the fingers, working from the nape area to the front hairline (j) & (k). Repeat the process once again if the hair needs to be straighter.

14   To check whether the hair is straight enough, remove some of the rearranger with a piece of cotton wool (l).

15   Once the hair is straight enough, rinse thoroughly and towel dry (m) & (n).

16   Apply winding lotion to the regrowth only, using a tinting bowl and brush or directly from the bottle if it has an applicator nozzle (o) & (p).

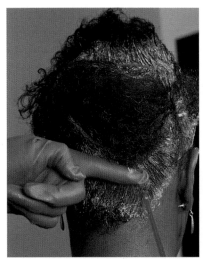
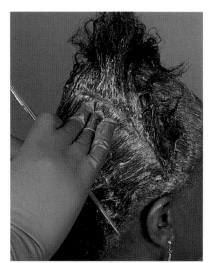
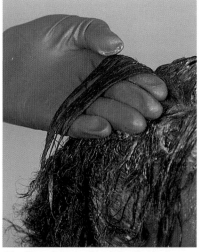

(j) & (k) Smoothing the regrowth area with the fingers

(l) Checking that the hair is rearranged sufficiently

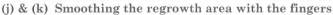

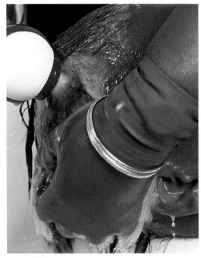
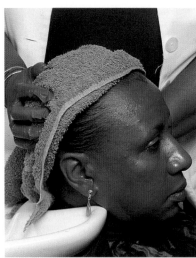
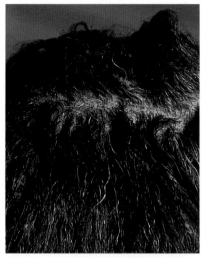

(m) Rinsing

(n) Towel-drying

The regrowth area after rearranger application

Tip

An 'S' curl will develop very quickly on African-Caribbean hair as the cuticle has already been opened by the rearranger.

17 After applying winding lotion, comb regrowth area only, starting from the nape and working up to the crown (q).

18 Start winding the hair from the back of the crown or from the front hairline, depending on where the most resistant part of the hair is. Continue winding the hair down to the nape (r).

19 Continue winding the hair from the front hairline to the top of the crown and sides until the whole head is wound (s).

20 Leave the hair to process with a plastic cap on, following the manufacturer's directions for timing. Processing time for most perms used on African-Caribbean hair is between 10 and 20 minutes (t).

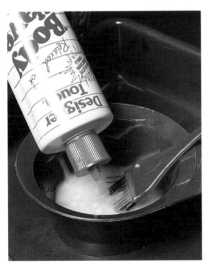

(o) Dispensing winding lotion into a bowl

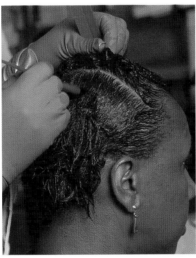

(p) Applying winding lotion to the regrowth

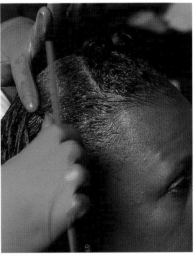

(q) Combing the regrowth area

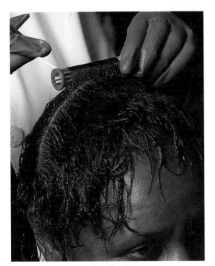

(r) Winding the hair

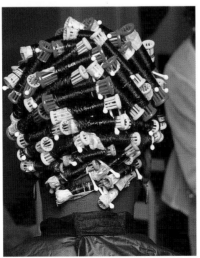

(s) The finished perm wind

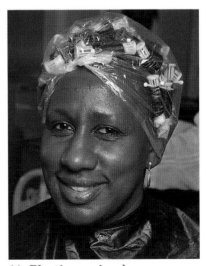

(t) Plastic cap in place

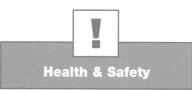

Health & Safety

Do not over-process the hair as this could weaken it and cause breakage.

21 After 10 minutes check for an 'S' curl by unwinding the rod or roller one and a half times. Gently push the hair upwards and look for an 'S' shape. Once this shape has developed look at a variety of perm rods throughout the head to ensure the required curl pattern has been achieved (u).

22 Once you are certain the hair has processed sufficiently, rinse thoroughly for 10 minutes (v).

23 Towel dry the hair and blot with cotton wool to remove excess water and avoid diluting the neutraliser (w) & (x).

24 Apply neutraliser recommended by the manufacturer. Leave neutraliser on with the rods in for the time instructed, which is usually 10 minutes. Make sure the neutraliser is left on for long enough, allowing the

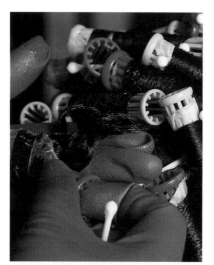

(u) Checking for 'S' curl

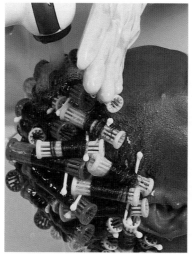

(v) Rinsing

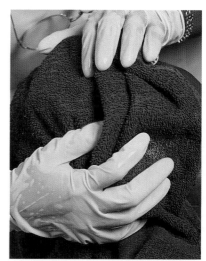

(w) Towel-drying

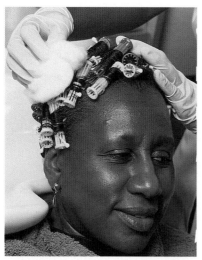

(x) Blotting excess water with cotton wool

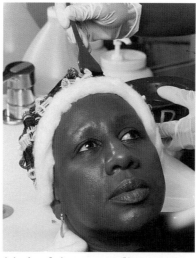

(y) Applying neutraliser

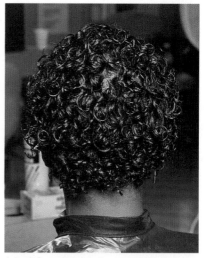

(z) After removing the rods

Tip

Always use conditioner on the hair after a perm as this will neutralise any traces of perm that may remain in the hair. Using a conditioner will restore the hair to its normal pH.

Tip

It is recommended that the hair is not set or blow-dried immediately after a perm, even if a perm product has been used which can be set or blow-dried. The hair should be naturally dried in its newly formed curl; it can be set on a follow-up visit to the salon.

chemical bonds in the hair to be reformed. This will also allow any perm lotion that might have been left in the hair to be neutralised (y).

25 Once the neutralising process has been completed, gently remove all rods (z). Rinse the hair thoroughly and apply a conditioner as recommended by the manufacturer.

26 Apply aftercare spray moisturiser and activator or the aftercare recommended by the perm product manufacturer – this will prevent the hair becoming dry and frizzy so that curls are more defined.

Tip

Neutraliser used on African-Caribbean hair usually contains Sodium Bromate. This has a more gentle action on the hair than peroxide-based neutraliser and leaves the hair in a better condition, but it takes longer to lock the new curl pattern into the hair. This is the reason why the rods remain in the hair throughout the neutralising process. Peroxide-based neutralisers are used on Caucasian hair, but are harsh when used on African-Caribbean hair. They also lighten the natural hair colour, making the hair reddish brown.

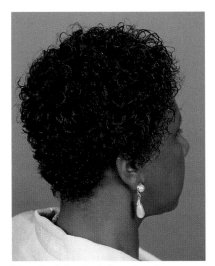

The finished style – back

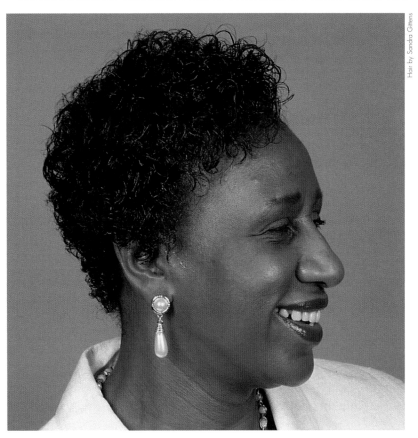

The finished style – side

Hair by Sandra Gittens

The chemical process is now complete. It is recommended that the hair is now cut into style. Once African-Caribbean hair has been permed it tends to be worn in its newly formed shape. If required, the hair can be set or blow-dried on a following visit to the salon. (For more information on aftercare see Chapter 6.)

Virgin hair application

Complete the preliminary procedures as outlined for regrowth perm application on page 127.

1   Shampoo the hair gently, taking care not to sensitise your client's scalp. Use the shampoo recommended by the product manufacturer. Remove excess moisture with a towel.

2   Apply a protective barrier around the hairline.

3   Apply pre-perm treatment to the ends if the mid-lengths and ends of the hair are porous and dry.

4   Apply rearranger to mid-lengths and ends first, as the ends will take longer to process. Start from the back of the hair working towards the front of the head.

5   Once you have applied rearranger throughout the mid-lengths and ends, begin applying rearranger to the root area, starting from the most resistant part. Cross check application for even coverage.

6   Put on a plastic cap and leave to process for 10–20 minutes, following manufacturer's instructions on timing.

7   Comb the hair gently, starting from the ends and working up through mid-lengths to roots, smoothing with the fingers. Repeat the process if necessary.

8   When the hair is straight enough, rinse thoroughly.

9   Starting at the nape and working up towards the front hairline, apply winding lotion to mid-lengths and ends then roots using a tinting brush or dispensing bottle. Comb the winding lotion through the hair.

10 Start winding from the middle of the crown, working backwards to the nape but leaving the crown and hairline until last.

11 Leave the hair to process with a plastic cap on. Follow manufacturer's directions for timing. The processing time for most perms used on African-Caribbean hair is between 10 and 20 minutes.

12 After the hair has been processed for 10 minutes or according to manufacturer's instructions, check for an

Tip

If the ends of the hair are in extremely good condition, do not apply any pre-perm treatment as this could form a barrier which would cause the hair to take longer to process.

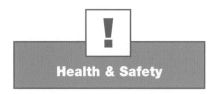

Health & Safety

Never use heat during the perming process unless stated by the manufacturer. Additional heat can cause severe damage to the scalp and hair.

Tip

When applying a chemical product to a virgin head of hair, always apply to the mid-lengths and ends first, working towards the root area. The hair nearer the scalp is warmer due to the heat from the head and this causes the hair to process more quickly. The further the hair is away from the scalp the longer it will take to process.

'S' curl by looking at a variety of perm rods throughout the head. If the curl pattern is not sufficient, check again every 5 minutes until the desired curl pattern is achieved. Rinse thoroughly for 10 minutes.

Follow steps 23 through to 26 in regrowth perm application.

Problems can develop during or after the perming process. The table outlines some problems, causes and solutions.

Problem	*Cause*	*Solution*
Hair frizzy after the perm	Hair not processed enough during the rearranging/straightening stage; incorrect strength perm used (product not strong enough)	Give a course of conditioning treatments if the hair cannot immediately take another perm. If the hair is in good condition, re-perm after two weeks; give a conditioning treatment in between perms.
Roots/regrowth frizzy, ends curly and smooth	Incorrect strength perm used; rearranger not left on long enough	Apply perm to regrowth only after giving the hair a course of conditioning treatment.
Curl drops after the perm	Rearranger product selected too strong or left on too long; hair has become over-processed	**Do not re-perm** – treat the hair until strong enough to perm. Cut the hair if necessary.
Curl drops after the perm	Hair not neutralised properly	Re-perm using winding lotion only; neutralise for the recommended time; **do not rearrange** the hair if it is straight enough.
Hair breaking after a perm	Hair damaged during the perming process (over-processed); chemical not rinsed out properly during the perming process	Give the hair a course of conditioning treatment; cut the hair if necessary.

Thermal styling

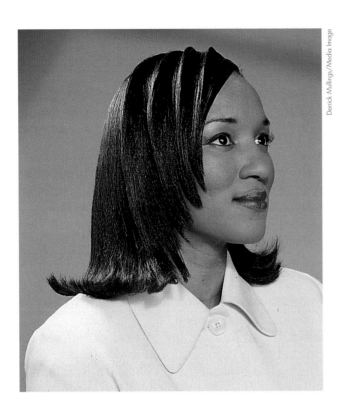

Derrick Mullings/Media Image

Learning objectives

This chapter covers the following:

- the science of thermal processing

- thermal styling products

- preparation of the hair prior to thermal styling

- use of thermal combs

- use of thermal tongs

Thermal styling of African-Caribbean hair is historically one of the first forms of processing the hair. It has been popular since the early nineteenth century when Madame C. J. Walker, an African American entrepreneur, produced the first pressing comb and hair care products for African-Caribbean hair. Thermal pressing and curling are only temporary processes and in the 1970s and 1980s became less popular, due to their poor durability in moist, humid conditions, which would make the hair revert to its natural curl (see Chapter 2 for more information on the hygroscopic property of hair). By the mid 1980s thermal styling had regained its popularity and was used to create a variety of different effects on the hair. Thermal styling was now being used on chemically processed hair to smooth and even out the cuticle.

Curling irons create a range of looks and shapes from curly, through wavy to smooth. The heat from the curling irons causes the curls formed and the finished style to be more durable. Although pressing combs have remained essentially the same over the years, curling tongs have evolved and are now manufactured in a variety of sizes and shapes.

Thermal styling can be a good option for the client whose hair is in a poor condition, or in need of a rest from chemical processing. It can be used on natural or relaxed hair. When thermal styling is used on natural hair it straightens out the curl temporarily. On chemically relaxed hair, thermal styling may be used to either straighten natural regrowth and even out the hair texture, or to smooth out unevenly relaxed hair.

Tip

Thermal processing is kinder to the hair than chemical processing.

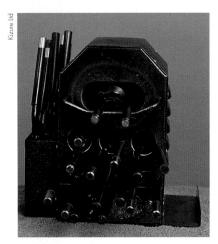

Kizure Ltd

Thermal styling heater with equipment

The science of thermal processing

Thermal processing is a physical rather than a chemical process. When the hair is thermally processed, water is removed from the hair. This is due to the heat produced by the thermal pressing comb or tong. The more water removed, the straighter the hair will remain and the longer the thermal process will last.

Hydrogen bonds are broken when the hair is pressed. The hotter the styling tools, the more hydrogen bonds are broken and a better, longer lasting result achieved (see Chapter 4 for more information). When natural hair is pressed or tonged it is a temporary process. The hair reverts back to its natural curl once moisture is absorbed from the atmosphere or the hair becomes wet.

Thermal styling products

There are many products on the market which are suitable for use when thermal styling. These products are of two types:

- pre-thermal styling sprays/lotions
- post-thermal styling sprays.

Pre-thermal styling sprays

These are used *before* thermal styling takes place. These products are applied to wet hair and protect the hair from the heat of the dryer or thermal styling tool. They contain conditioners and polymers which coat and protect the hair during processing. The hair is then blow dried or allowed to dry naturally. Thermal processing can then take place.

Post-thermal styling sprays

These are hair lacquers and consist of a synthetic, adhesive polymer dissolved in alcohol to give hold. They may also contain small amounts of conditioning agents. They are sprayed onto the finished style to create a solid, firm finish and protect the hair against atmospheric conditions. Post-thermal styling sprays can be used on the hair *prior* to tonging to protect it from the heat of the tongs and create a crisp, smoothly defined curl.

Preparation of the hair prior to thermal styling

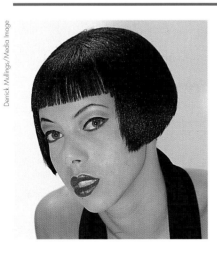

Derrick Mullings/Media Image

Prior to any thermal styling being carried out, a thorough consultation and analysis should be given and the hair must be shampooed and conditioned. Failure to cleanse the hair properly can result in unpleasant odours and smoke during the thermal processing caused by the burning of residues on the hair. (For further information on selecting a suitable shampoo and conditioner, see Chapter 3.)

Consultation

1 Examine the client's scalp and hair.
2 Discuss with your client the result to be achieved.
3 Discuss any concerns she may have about the process to be carried out.

Tip

Never thermally process dirty hair as this could cause the hair to become damaged and break.

Analysis

1   Assess the natural curl in the hair, its texture, condition and density. This will help you decide on the degree of straightness required.
2   Decide which shampoo and conditioning treatment should be used.
3   Select the thermal styling products to be used.
4   Select the thermal styling technique to be used.

Use of thermal combs

Thermal combs come in a variety of shapes and sizes. Some have a curved back for added smoothness. Some have widely spread teeth for thicker, coarser hair; others have closer set teeth for finer hair. Like the choice of a pair of cutting scissors, the selection of thermal styling tools is made essentially on their ability to do the job at hand and the personal choice of the stylist.

Thermal combs are of two types, **electrical** and **non-electrical**:

- **Non-electrical combs** tend to be hotter than electrical pressing combs. These combs are heated to a high temperature in a special electrical heater. Before using the comb on the hair, its temperature must be checked and if necessary it must be first cooled on a thermal cooling pad.

- **Electrical combs** are plugged into the mains and the temperature is controlled by a thermostat built into the comb. The disadvantage of using electrical pressing combs is that the element can burn out, also the temperature tends to be lower and may not be sufficient to straighten the hair effectively.

Equipment needed for thermal pressing

- pressing comb
- thermal heating stove (if using a non-electrical pressing comb)
- de-tangling comb
- water spray
- thermal cooling pad (to control the heat of the pressing comb)
- tissue paper.

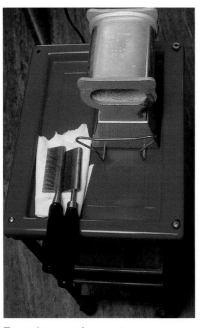

Pressing equipment

Safe use of thermal pressing combs

1   Select a suitable pressing comb depending on the thickness of the hair.

2   Check the temperature of the pressing comb before attempting to press the hair. To test the temperature of the comb, place it on a tissue. If the tissue becomes scorched or burns the comb is too hot.

3   If the pressing comb is too hot, cool electrical pressing combs by reducing the temperature – never spray water on them. When working with non-electrical pressing combs, cool the comb by placing it on a cooling pad. If necessary spray with water.

- Place the thermal pressing comb 12.5 mm (half an inch) away from the scalp to avoid burning.
- Always hold the hair at a 45 degree angle to avoid burning the scalp with the pressing comb.
- Use the back of the pressing comb to straighten the hair.

Pressing technique

1   Gown and protect the client.

2   Carry out a thorough consultation and analysis.

3   Prepare the hair by applying the correct shampoo and conditioning treatment (see Chapter 3).

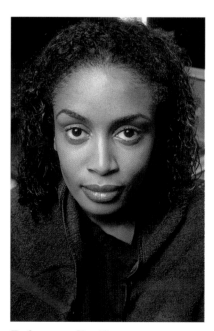

Before application

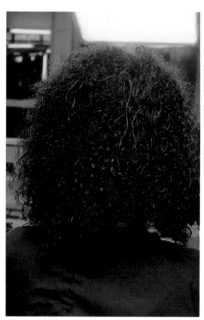

Back view of natural hair prior to pressing

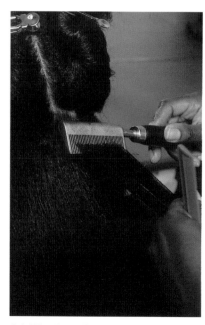

(a) Placing the comb into the hair half an inch away from the scalp

4   Select a suitable drying technique for the hair (see Chapter 5).

5   De-tangle the hair and divide into four sections.

6   Sub-divide the hair into a 6 mm (quarter of an inch) section starting at the nape

7   After testing the temperature, place the teeth of the pressing comb 12.5 mm (half an inch) away from the scalp in a upwards position, pressing the underneath of the hair first.

8   Pull the pressing comb through the roots, mid-lengths and ends of the hair (a), (b) & (c).

9   Press the same section of hair on top to finish the process. Turn the wrist outwards, away from you. Use the back of the comb to straighten the hair. Feed the hair slowly through the comb as you work down towards the ends of the hair (d).

10   Continue the straightening process throughout the hair using the same technique.

11   Stand in front of the client to gently press around the front hairline.

Process the hair according to the hair texture and the kind of look you would like to achieve. For example, when working on natural hair, repeat the above process so that the hair is pressed twice. This will give a straighter look. When chemically relaxed hair is being pressed to smooth out the cuticle, the process should be carried out only once.

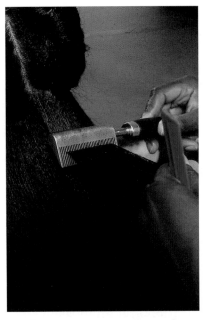

(b) Taking the comb through the hair

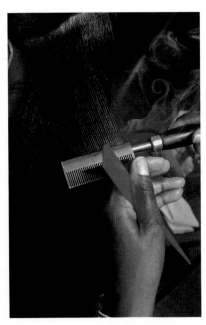

(c) Continuing to press the section of hair

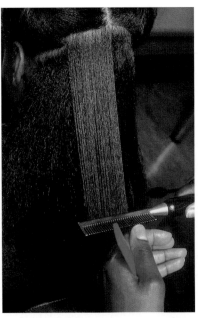

(d) Using the back of the comb to press and smooth the section of hair

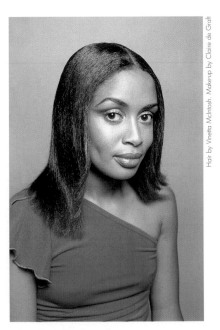

The finished style

Hair by Vinetta McIntosh. Makeup by Claire de Graft

Use of thermal tongs

Tip

Prior to thermal pressing it is better to blow-dry the hair using the blow-dry attachment or comb technique. This will smooth the natural curl in preparation for thermal pressing (see Chapter 5).

Tip

To avoid burning the scalp, always make sure the hair is completely dry before attempting any thermal processing.

Health & Safety

It is best to apply dressing to the scalp after the hair has been thermally pressed, rather than during the pressing process, otherwise the heat of the comb combined with the dressing could scald the scalp.

Tip

Before using the pressing comb, test the temperature on tissue or a cooling pad. Make sure the temperature is correct by testing on the ends of the hair first.

Thermal tongs, like thermal combs, are available in a variety of shapes and sizes. The size of tong selected is dependent on the length of the hair and the style to be achieved. A variety of curl shapes can be produced by tonging:

- waves
- barrel curls
- spiral curls
- root curls
- off-base/dragged curls.

Using professional tongs proficiently and correctly comes only with practice and experience. Before attempting to use tongs, particularly those with swivel handles, it is important to learn to control and use them correctly.

The correct way to hold electrical tongs

There are two basic movements used to control the tongs:

- opening and closing the barrel
- turning the tongs.

Opening and closing the barrel

1 Hold the tong upright with the thicker end of the barrel at the bottom.
2 Place the first three fingers on the outside of the handle.
3 Place the thumb on the inside of the handle nearest to you.
4 Place the tip of the little finger on the lower handle so that it is pointing in towards you.
5 Open and close the fingers using the little finger to control the movement.

This action will produce a clicking sound with the tongs and enables the hair to move smoothly through the barrel.

Once you have mastered this, move on to the next stage.

Tip

Opening and closing the tongs will allow the hair to move freely while tonging; turning the tongs allows a curl to be achieved.

Turning the tongs

Try rotating the tongs, turning the handles inwards and towards you. This action enables a curl to be formed. Practise this movement until you are comfortable with it. The correct use of the tongs involves a combination of these two movements.

Curling tongs can be **electrical** or **non-electrical**.

- **Electrical tongs** have a thermostat built into them which controls the temperature. They are kinder to the hair as they do not become as hot as non-electrical tongs. However, because of this the type of styles that can be achieved are limited. The disadvantage of using this type of tong is that the end result is not as durable as with non-electrical tongs. Electrical tongs do not come in such a wide variety of shapes and sizes as non-electrical tongs.

- **Non-electrical tongs** can get much hotter, allowing the stylist to achieve a greater variety of effects. The hotter the tongs, the greater will be the durability of the finished style. For this reason they must be used with additional care, observing the correct safety precautions as outlined earlier in this chapter for non-electrical pressing combs. Non-electrical tongs are available in a wide variety of shapes and sizes.

Equipment needed for thermal tonging

- tongs
- thermal heating stove (if non-electrical tongs used)
- de-tangling comb
- tail comb
- water spray
- thermal cooling pad (to control the heat of the tongs)
- tissue.

Safe use of thermal, non-electrical tongs

1 Select the size of tongs to be used according to the length of the hair and the style to be achieved.

2 Check the temperature of the tongs before attempting to tong the hair. Test the temperature by placing them on a tissue. If the tissue becomes scorched or burns the tongs are too hot. Place extremely hot tongs on a cooling pad and spray with water.

3 Always smooth the root area of the hair by placing the tongs at the roots. Grip the hair and pull the tong down the hair shaft a few times, then place the tongs in the desired position for tonging. This will do two things – smooth the cuticle and establish a firm grip on the hair with the tongs.

4 When creating root curls or barrel curls, hold the hair at a 90° angle when tonging.

5 When creating dragged curls, hold the hair at a 45° angle when tonging.

6 For added protection and if you are unsure, place a comb under the tongs to protect the scalp, especially when working on short hair. This will allow you to get closer to the scalp.

Tonging techniques

Barrel curl

Barrel curls produce a soft, open-ended curl ideal for styles which require a softer, freer look, or support after wrap-setting or blow-drying.

1 Take a section of hair and smooth the roots between the two barrels of the tongs (a).

2 Pull the tongs to the ends of the hair, maintaining an even tension.

3 When you reach the ends of the hair, wind the tongs up to the roots. Maintain tension to avoid the ends slipping out of the tongs (b) & (c).

4 At the root area, open and close the tongs to free the ends of the hair. Hold the tongs in place for a few seconds to develop a firm, smooth, even curl (d).

5 Rotate the tongs within the newly formed curl to free the points of the hair (e).

6 Gently remove the tongs (f).

Tip

Place a comb under the tongs when working near the root area to avoid burning the scalp.

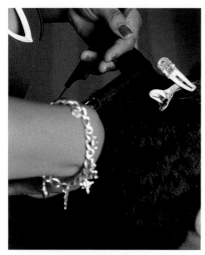

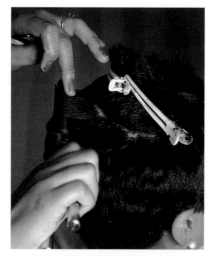

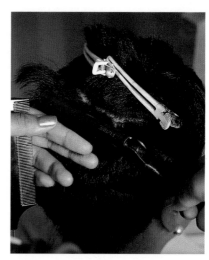

(a) Smoothing the roots   (b) & (c) Winding the tongs to the roots

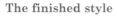

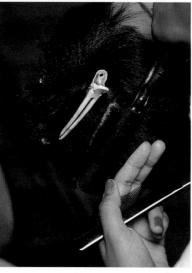

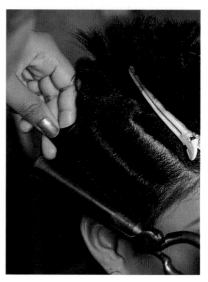

(d) Holding the tongs in place
with the comb inside acting as
a guard to protect the scalp

(e) Rotating the tongs to free
the ends

(f) Gently removing the tongs

The finished style

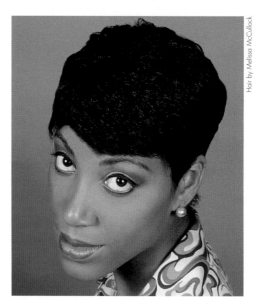

Hair by Melissa McCullock

Spiral tonging

This technique is suitable for shoulder-length hair and longer. It produces vertical curls that cascade downwards, forming a spiral/ringlet effect.

1   Section the hair in nine sections (as for perming). Take a vertical section 25 mm (1 inch) in length, starting at the nape of the neck.
2   Work from left to right.
3   Place the tongs 12 mm (half an inch) away from the scalp. Smooth the roots of the hair with the tongs.
4   Turn the strand of hair to be tonged inwards towards the left.
5   Open and close the barrel to feed the hair through.
6   Continue to wind the hair down the barrel of the tong, opening and closing the barrel to release the hair through.
7   When you reach the ends of the hair, rotate the barrel to ensure the ends of the hair are curled.

Off-base tonging

This technique is ideal when movement is required on the ends of the hair. The hair is tonged at a 45° angle throughout the head and produces dragged curls with no root movement. The hair can be tonged in an upwards or downwards position.

Off-base tonging long, layered hair

This technique is ideal for creating styles where the ends of the hair will be flipped upwards.

1   Smooth the hair along the roots between the two barrels of the tong (a).
2   Pull the tongs to the ends of the hair, maintaining an even tension. When you reach the ends of the hair, start winding the hair upwards, turning the ends under (b).
3   Hold the tong in position and allow the curl to be formed. Rotate the tong inside the hair to free the ends. Remove the tongs gently (c).

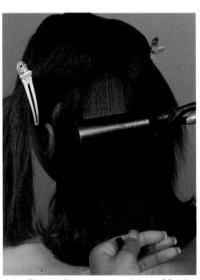
(a) Smoothing a section of hair

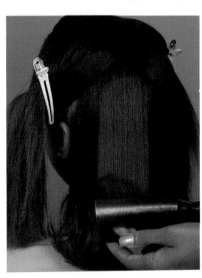
(b) Winding the ends of the hair

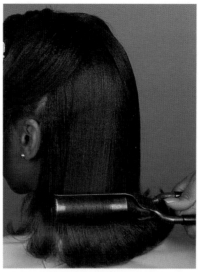

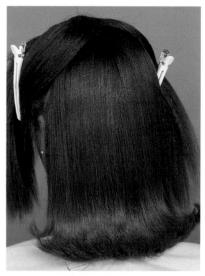

(c) Holding the tongs at the ends to create movement

The hair after tonging

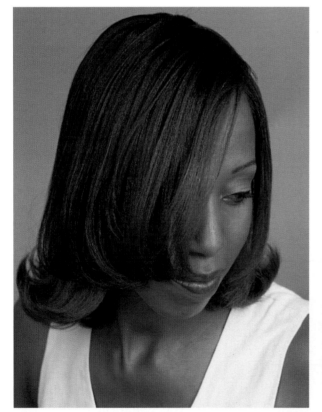

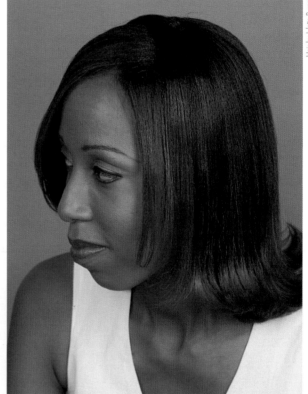

Hair by Juliette Burnett

The finished hairstyle

Off-base tonging a short, graduated hairstyle

This technique is ideal for styles where the ends of the hair need to be curled under.

1   Start tonging the hair from the back, smoothing the hair along the roots between the two barrels of the tong and curling the ends of the hair under (a) & (b). Follow the same procedure as in step 3 on page 147 (c).

2   Proceed onto the sides (d).

3   Work up to the crown of the head and tong the front of the hair.

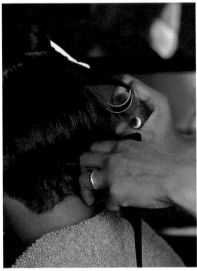

(a) Smoothing a section of hair

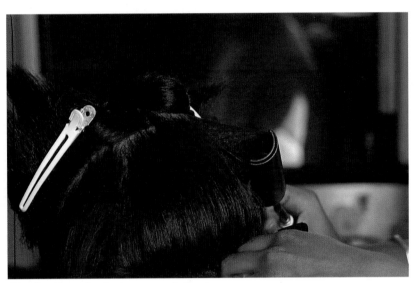

(b) Curling the hair around the tongs

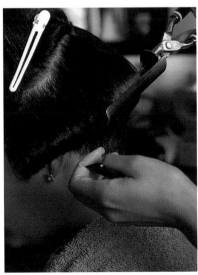

(c) Allowing the curl to form on the ends before gently removing it

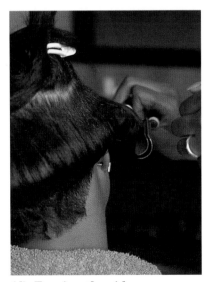

(d) Tonging the sides

The finished hair style after tonging

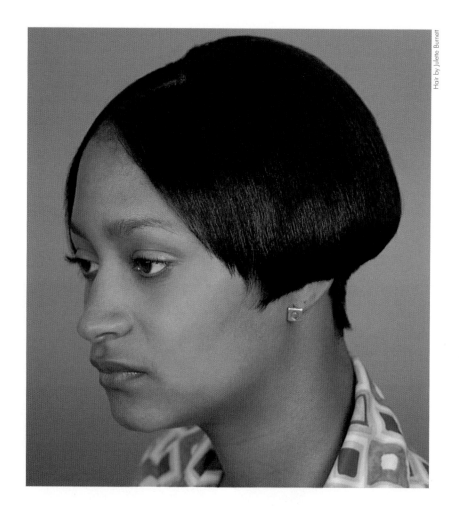

Hair by Julelie Burnett

Cutting

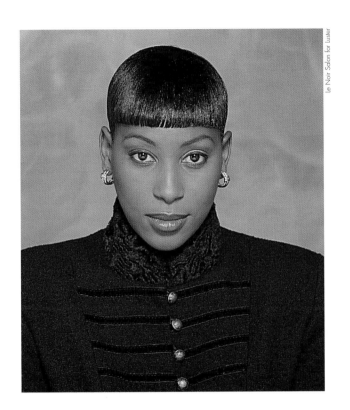

Le Noir Salon for Luster

Learning objectives

This chapter covers the following:

- **cutting tools, cutting terminology and techniques**
- **natural movement and hair growth patterns**
- **outline shapes**
- **consultation and analysis**
- **inverted one-length cut, graduated cut and layered cut**
- **long layered/over-directed cut**
- **fashion cut**
- **sculpture cut**

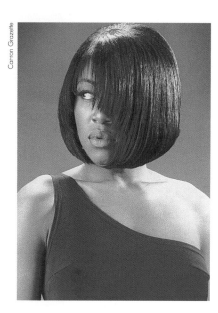

Carron Grazette

A good hair cut is the basis for achieving any hairstyle. Cutting the hair into style allows the hairdresser to show his/her creativity – when we cut hair we are using it as a medium to design and create an overall look for the client.

As hairdressers, it is important that our cutting skills are as good as all the other services we carry out within the salon. A good haircut can totally transform a head of hair. To be able to create the right effect and be technically correct you need to be able to execute a number of different hair-cutting techniques. You must also have a knowledge of face shapes, hair texture, movement and direction, all of which must be taken into consideration prior to carrying out any haircut.

It is essential to have a knowledge of basic cutting techniques before attempting to cut anyone's hair. Knowledge and experience can be gained through watching demonstrations and videos, and practising on tuition heads and models. Practice will help you develop technically along with developing the art of hair control.

Over the years hairdressers and large salon groups have developed their own terminology for describing various cutting techniques. These techniques have not changed throughout the history of hairdressing and regardless of terminology used they create the same effect. There are three basic cutting techniques that can be achieved when cutting hair:

- **layering**
- **graduation**
- **one-length shapes**.

Basic cuts and shapes can be totally changed by texturising, tailoring or personalising a cut to suit the client's lifestyle, requirements, face shape and hair texture. Fashion is constantly revolving. Each time a style becomes fashionable again the basic style remains but is updated to reflect current fashion trends.

There are many reasons for cutting hair:

- to enhance the shape
- to make the hair manageable
- to design a new shape
- to remove damaged hair.

Regardless of the hair type, the basic techniques of cutting hair are the same. When working with African-Caribbean hair, allowances must be made for natural movement within the hair. Always use even tension when cutting

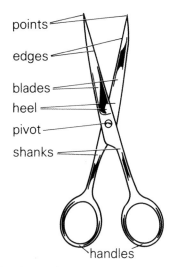

points
edges
blades
heel
pivot
shanks
handles

Cutting scissors

Tip

Before purchasing a pair of cutting scissors, try out a few pairs for comfort, length and weight.

Tip

Hairdressing scissors should be regularly set and re-sharpened to maintain their sharpness.

!

Health & Safety

Cleanse scissors with methylated spirits after normal use. If you accidentally cut the skin, the scissors should be sterilised in an autoclave or a sterilising solution which will not cause the scissors to rust. (For further information see Chapter 15.)

naturally curly hair; this will help you to stretch and control the hair during cutting. Always cut the hair slightly longer than the intended length as the hair will appear shorter when dry.

Cutting tools

Cutting scissors

Hairdressing scissors are made up of two blades fastened with a screw which acts as a pivot. The diagram details the parts of a pair of cutting scissors.

Before even attempting to cut a head of hair, the correct tools must be selected. When choosing scissors you should take into account their weight, their length and most importantly how comfortable they feel in your hands. Scissors can range from the fairly cheap to the very expensive. The more you pay for scissors, the better the quality and more accurate the cut.

The correct way to hold a pair of cutting scissors is between the thumb and third finger. Holding the scissors in this way will give the best control and balance. The action used when cutting is the opening and closing of the scissors using the thumb only. When cutting hair, use the middle to the points of your blades. Work through the hair in small precise bites for control.

Thinning scissors

Thinning scissors are used to remove bulk and weight from the hair. They are of two types:

- Those with notched teeth on the cutting edge of both blades – these scissors will remove maximum bulk or weight from the hair.
- Those with notched teeth on the cutting edge of one blade only; the other blade has a straight cutting edge – these scissors will remove minimum bulk and weight from the hair.

Cutting combs

Cutting combs vary in size and the choice very much depends on the stylist selecting the comb with which he/she is most comfortable. Sometimes a larger tooth comb is better, for example when working on a thicker head of hair.

Tip

Take care of your scissors. Only use them for cutting hair. If hairdressing scissors are used for cutting paper or cloth it could damage the cutting edge, making the scissors dull and no longer suitable for cutting hair.

Health & Safety

On completion of a haircut, any combs used should be washed in soapy water, rinsed and placed in a suitable sterilising solution. (For further information see Chapter 15.)

A more flexible comb is better for scissors-over-comb work when cutting the hair very short in the nape area. When sculpture cutting the hair, an Afro comb is best for controlling the hair lengths and following the contours of the head.

Natural movement and hair growth patterns

All curly hair has natural movement but this is not always seen clearly on very curly hair due to its dense appearance. Natural curl or movement is more commonly seen in relaxed or wavy hair. When we refer to natural movement we are describing any extreme changes in how the hair grows. The following table outlines hair growth patterns.

Growth Pattern	Where Found	How to deal with it
Widow's peak	Prominent point found at the front hairline	The hair tends to work best when styled backwards; fringes are best kept long to avoid spiking.
Double crown	Two circular movements found on the crown and further back on the head on opposite sides	Found on wavier hair; leave the hair longer in these areas to avoid spiking.
Nape whirls	Found in the nape; strong circular movement on either side of the head	The hair needs to be left slightly longer so it will remain flat; alternatively cut the hair very close to the scalp to avoid spiking.
Cow's lick	Strong movement in the front hairline directing the hair to the right or left; found in straight and wavy hair	Always cut hair in the same direction in which it naturally falls. Leave weight on fringes to avoid spiking and make the hair lie flatter.

Cutting terminology and techniques

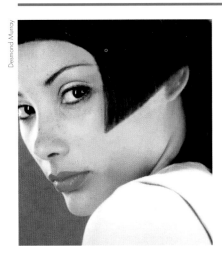

Before attempting to cut a head of hair, a knowledge of cutting terminology is useful. Terminology used varies within the hairdressing industry but the technique remains the same.

Terminology

analysis stylist looks at natural growth pattern, movement and decides on techniques to be used and the look to be achieved

asymmetric one side of the hair is cut longer than the other

blending technique that describes the continuation or blending of one section of the haircut into another

channel cutting working in lines throughout the haircut

consultation discussion between client and stylist on look to be achieved, manageability and aftercare

crown top middle section of the head

external shape the perimeter of the haircut

fashion cutting using a combination of cutting techniques to create a fashion look

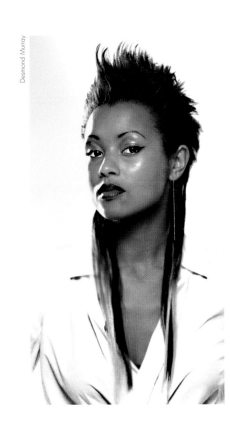

free hand cutting cutting the hair without tension – not holding the hair during the cutting process

guideline first section of hair cut to establish length and shape to be achieved

hairline hair growth framing the outside of the head nearest the face and neck

horseshoe section hair sectioned from the crown to the front hairline in a horseshoe shape

internal guideline the first section of hair cut to determine the internal shape

internal shape the internal/inner shape of the haircut

mesh sub-division or smaller piece of hair taken from the main section

nape back section of the head at the hairline near the neck

occipital bone the bone that sits between each ear, sometimes identified by a prominent bump

sculpture cut cut following the contours of the head

sectioning dividing the hair into manageable sections prior to cutting

symmetric both sides of the haircut are the same length

tension the amount of stretch placed on the hair during cutting

weight length and bulk of the hair

Cutting techniques

club cutting produces a solid blunt line – this can make the hair appear thicker

graduated cut the hair is held away from the scalp at a 45° angle and cut – this creates layers on the perimeter of the hair

layer cut hair cut at various angles to create layers and movement within a haircut

one-length cut hair cut on the perimeter only

over-directed technique used to create length and weight on the perimeter of the hair with shorter layers internally

scissors-over-comb cutting the hair close to the scalp using scissors or clippers over a comb

Texturising techniques

Texturising is the removal of weight from the hair using a variety of techniques. The points of the hair are left thinner. This technique is ideal for breaking up solid lines.

The following techniques are used when texturising the hair:

pointing the points of the scissors are used to snip into the hair at intervals along the hair strands to break up solid lines and create texture

serrating the blunt edges of the hair are broken up by chipping into it with the points of the scissors

slicing/slither cutting the scissors are glided through meshes of hair, taking away length and bulk

twist-texturising sections of the hair are twisted and the scissors run up and down the hair, removing length and bulk

Outline shapes

Different shapes can be created on the perimeter of a cut, regardless of the length of the hair. Different shapes and angles can create hard or soft lines. For example, a solid straight line can create a hard finish. Softer lines can be created by texturising, layering or graduating the hair.

Short shape outlines

Before changing the outline shape on the perimeter of the hair, the shape of the client's head, neck and hairline must be taken into consideration. Cutting the hair following the client's natural growth pattern can create a softer finish, particularly when creating short looks on female clients.

Designing perimeter shapes

Tip

If the hair is cut against the skin it creates a hard shape. If the hair is cut away from the skin a softer look will be achieved.

Different outlines can be created on the perimeter by using the techniques described below. Always remember that the angle and direction at which you hold the hair will determine the effect and shape created. For example, the lower the fingers are held (a), the less graduation will be achieved; the higher the fingers are held (b) the more graduation will be achieved.

If the fingers are sloped or angled in a downward position, the hair will be cut shorter at one point and longer at another. This will encourage the hair to move forwards and

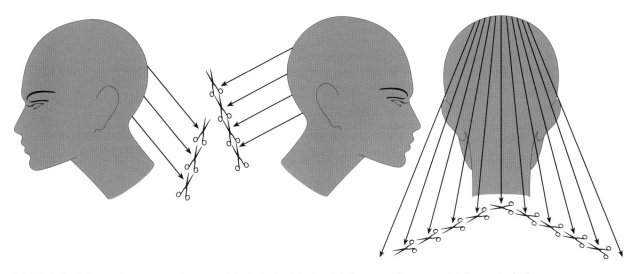

(a) Hair held at a lower angle   (b) Hair held at a higher angle   (c) Inverted shape

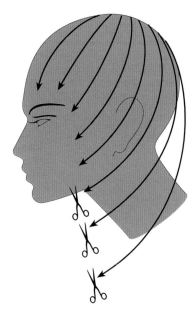

(d) Page boy

Tip

Fringes can be layered to create fullness and softness or cut to one length to create a solid, straight line.

Tip

Discuss with your client the length they would like their fringe to be. This will avoid the hair being cut too short.

Tip

Try to avoid cutting fringes too short as they can become spiky and unnatural, unless this is the effect you wish to create.

create weight where the length has built up. For example an inverted bob (c).

When the fingers are sloped or angled in an upward position, the opposite will take place. The hair will be shorter at one point and longer at another. This technique will push the weight away from the front to the back of the hair where it is longer. For example a page boy style (d) or feathered cut.

Cutting a fringe

A fringe can add variety and interest to a hairstyle but will not suit all clients. It can vary in length, thickness and texture. The choice of the type of fringe to be worn will depend on the hairstyle, client requirements, hair texture and creativity of the stylist.

A fringe can be cut using a variety of shapes such as:

- **curved** – ideal for clients who like the hair to frame the forehead and sides of the hairline. This will produce softer lines.
- **square** – will produce a hard, geometric, solid line.
- **triangular** – ideal for creating a thicker, fuller fringe. This type of fringe can be layered to give more volume and softness.

When cutting a fringe, cut the hair without using too much tension or cut it freehand, allowing the hair to fall naturally while cutting. Using this technique will stop the hair from springing up and sticking out. Once you have decided on the shape of fringe you want to create, proceed as follows.

1 Sub-divide the hair, starting at the front hairline.
2 Bring down sections of hair, cutting to the guideline.
3 Cut to the thickness required. (If required, layer-cut the hair once all the hair has been cut to a solid length.)
4 Cross check the fringe to ensure it is even.

Consultation and analysis

Before a cut is carried out, the following details concerning the client need to be taken into account:

- lifestyle
- head and face shape
- hair texture and movement
- requirements
- the look to be achieved.

Lifestyle

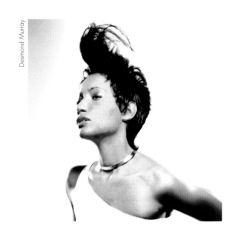

You must consider your client's job, interests and hobbies. It is important to find out how active a lifestyle your client leads as this will help you to plan a suitable cut. For example, if your client is involved with sports on a regular basis, a style which needs minimum maintenance would be best.

Head and face shape

It is important to take into consideration the client's head and face shape prior to cutting the hair. Your observations will help you to decide on a suitable style and shape for the client. (For further information see Chapter 1.)

Hair texture

Prior to cutting, you must look at the client's hair texture as certain cuts will be more suitable for particular textures. For example, fine hair cut in a one-length style will appear thicker.

In African-Caribbean hair, tighter curled textures show little or no movement. However, when the hair has been relaxed or sculpture cut, natural movement is more apparent. In wavy textured African-Caribbean hair, natural partings and texture are more prevalent and more easily defined than in curly hair. A variety of hair growth patterns can be seen such as nape whirls, widow's peak, double crown and cow's lick. All these growth patterns must be taken into consideration prior to cutting.

Tip

Nothing looks worse than hair cut short in the nape which does not complement the client's hair growth pattern or neck.

Client requirements

Remember that your client is part of the cutting process so should be involved in the look to be achieved. After considering all the above you should now be in a better position to decide on the cut and shape to be achieved.

Discuss in depth with your client the style you are going to create. Make sure she agrees and is happy with the changes you are going to make to her hair. It is important that she is not only happy with the cut but will be able to manage the finished look. Advice must be given on how the cut and shape is to be maintained. Before even attempting to cut a head of hair you must be sure of your client's ability to maintain the new look. There is no point in giving a client a new style which she will not be able to maintain at home.

The look to be achieved

Once you have reached agreement with your client on the cut to be achieved, you can proceed. Following all the above guidelines will avoid any complications arising during or after the haircut. The finished style should suit the client and work in harmony with the hair texture, face shape, natural movement and lifestyle.

Inverted one-length cut (bob)

Tip

When cutting a one-length bob, the guideline on the perimeter of the hair in the nape area can be cut straight or with an inverted shape (sometimes called an A shape). If the hair is cut straight, when the head is held in an upright position a curved outline will be produced on the perimeter. The reverse happens if the hair is cut with an inversion – the outline on the perimeter is straight when the head is held upright.

A one-length cut creates weight on the perimeter, with no internal movement. It is important that all meshes of hair are cut to the same length to create an even and balanced finish. If you cut the hair close to the skin you will create a 0° angle. Cutting the hair between the fingers will produce a 45° angle. A classic bob is a good example of a one-length hair cut.

Procedure for cutting an inverted bob

1 Gown and protect the client.
2 Carry out a consultation and analysis with the client.
3 Shampoo and condition the client's hair.
4 Divide the hair into four sections and sub-divide the two nape sections. This should be no thicker than 6 mm ($\frac{1}{4}$ inch) (a).
5 Start cutting the guideline on the left side first, holding the fingers in a downwards sloping position. Hold the fingers parallel to the section (b) & (c).

Tip

Do not use too much tension as you work on the sides over the ears. Protruding ears could cause the hair to spring up in this area and become shorter than the rest of the cut.

6 Proceed towards the right side of the head, sloping or angling the fingers in the opposite direction. This will create an inverted shape (d) & (e).

7 Continue cutting the hair to the initial guideline, holding the hair at a 45° angle (f) & (g).

8 As you work up the hair, gradually straighten the section.

9 Continue to proceed up the head, taking 6 mm ($\frac{1}{4}$ inch) sections and working left to right until you reach the crown (h).

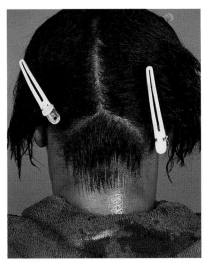

(a) The hair sectioned prior to cutting

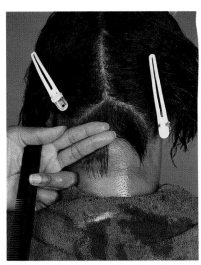

(b) Two fingers showing the cutting angle

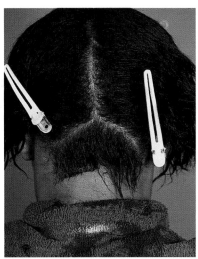

(c) The first section of the guideline after cutting

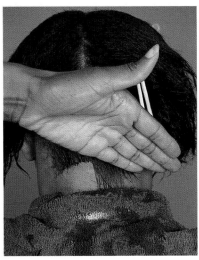

(d) Angling the fingers on the right

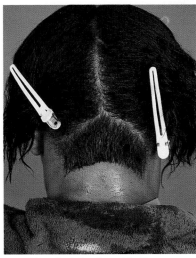

(e) The finished guideline

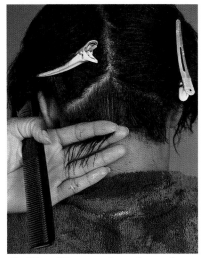

(f) Blending sections into the guideline and cutting

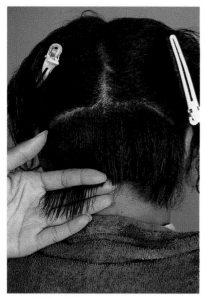

(g) Working through the head, cutting to the guideline

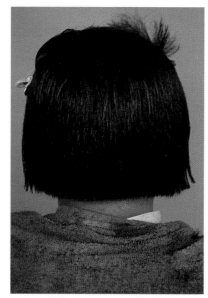

(h) The finished cut at the back

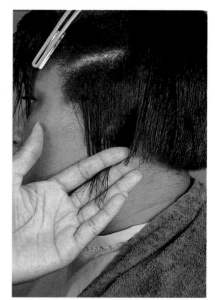

(i) Establishing the left side guideline

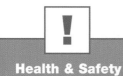

Health & Safety

Avoid walking around the salon with open scissors as this could cause unnecessary accidents. When scissors are not in use, leave them closed and in their pouch.

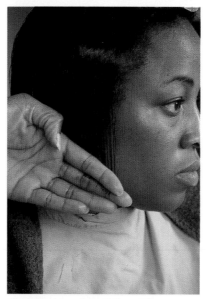

(j) Cutting the right side guideline

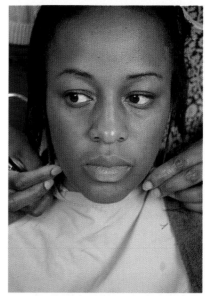

(k) Checking that both sides have been cut evenly

Tip

Cutting the hair with a centre parting will ensure that the cut is symmetrical. The hair can then be worn with a side parting, middle parting or swept back. If the client is going to wear her hair only with a side parting, cut the hair with a side parting instead of a middle parting. This will create weight and length on the side of the parting. The hair will now have to be worn permanently with a side parting as the cut will not be symmetrical.

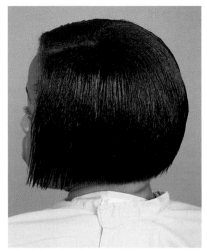

The finished cut

Tip

Use parts of the face –
ears, nose, chin – to
measure and balance the
length of hair when
cutting.

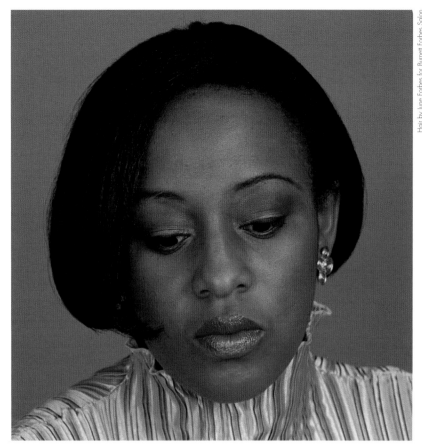

The finished style after blow-drying and tonging

Tip

To ensure that the hair is
cut to the same length on
both sides, measure your
guideline against the side
already cut. Once the two
sides are the same
continue cutting.

10   Proceed to the left side of the head. Sub-divide the hair
     taking 6 mm ($\frac{1}{4}$ inch) sections. Blend the back section to
     the side, angling the fingers downwards to create a
     sloped effect on the sides. This will establish your side
     guideline (i).

11   Follow the same procedure on the right side of the
     head (j).

12   Check that both sides of the haircut are equal (k).

Graduated cut

This cut creates layers and weight on the perimeter of the
hair. The layers can be high or low depending on the result
to be achieved.

Procedure for graduated cut

1   Follow steps 1 to 3 for an inverted bob on page 160.

2   Divide the hair into four sections. Sub-divide the hair in 6 mm ($\frac{1}{4}$ inch) sections at the nape. Cut the guideline close to the neck at a 0° angle (a).

3   Take three sub-divisions of hair down until a solid line is formed in the nape area (b).

4   Blend the hair in the nape area by layering at a 90° angle (c).

5   Take a horizontal sub-section of hair and create the internal guideline by cutting the hair at a 45° angle. Do not lift the hair higher than the ears when graduating at this angle (d).

6   Make sure the hair is combed from roots to ends to ensure that the hair is cut evenly. When the back of the hair is completely cut, proceed to the sides.

7   Establish the side guideline and blend to the back guideline. Once a solid line has been developed, start lifting the hair using the same technique as before so that graduation is developed throughout the perimeter (e).

8   Repeat the process on the opposite side of the head.

9   Cut the fringe area and blend to both sides (f) & (g).

10   Cross check the cut.

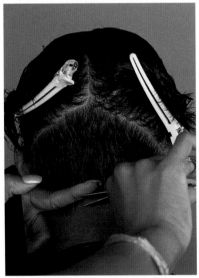

(a) Cutting the guideline close to the neck

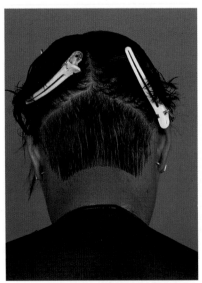

(b) A solid line after cutting three sub-divisions

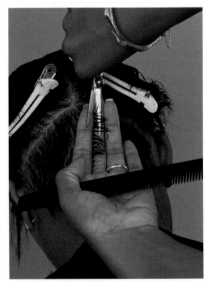

(c) Blending the nape area by cutting at a 90° angle

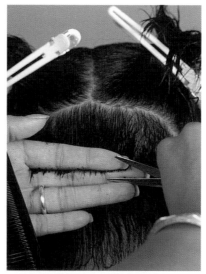

(d) Creating the internal guideline

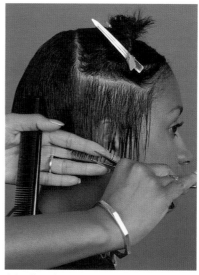

(e) Cutting the right side guideline

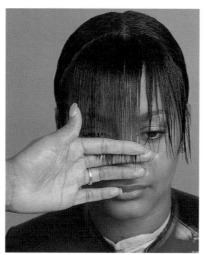

(f) Cutting the fringe

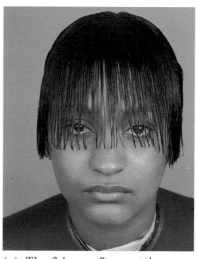

(g) The fringe after cutting

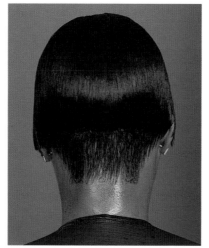

The finished wet cut – back

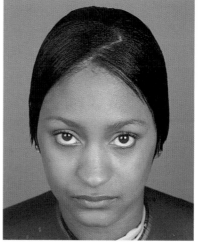

The finished wet cut – front

The finished style after blow-drying and tonging

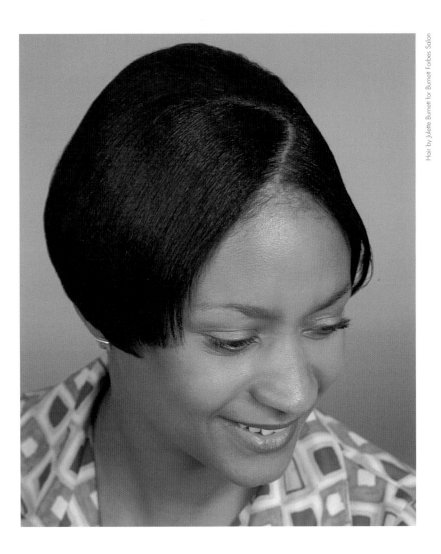

Hair by Juliette Burnett for Burnett Forbes Salon

Short layered cut

A uniform layer is cut at a 90° angle. Length is removed internally throughout the cut. All sections of hair are cut to the same length, following the contours of the head.

Procedure for short layered cut

1   Follow steps 1 to 3 for an inverted bob on page 160.
2   Divide the hair into six sections (a).
3   Starting at the nape, sub-divide the hair taking 6 mm ($\frac{1}{4}$ inch) sections (b). Cut the guideline at a 0° angle (c).
4   Continue to take sub-sections down, cutting the hair to the original guideline until a solid line is formed (d).
5   Take a vertical section from the nape to the occipital bone or just below the ears (e).

6   Hold the hair at a 90° angle and cut. Work from left to right, holding the hair at the same angle until you reach the crown (f).

7   Proceed to the sides. Cut the perimeter guideline at a 45° angle (g).

8   Continue cutting the hair at a 90° angle throughout the sides. Cut the other side of the hair using the same technique (h) & (i).

9   Start cutting the horseshoe section horizontally until you reach the front hairline (j).

10 Cross check the whole cut, checking in the opposite direction to the direction in which the hair was cut. For example, if the hair was cut by taking horizontal sections, cross check with vertical sections and vice versa.

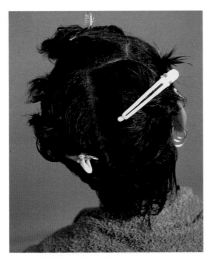

(a) The hair sectioned into six

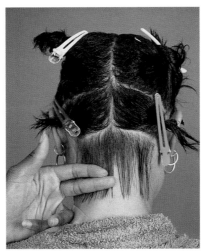

(b) Sub-division of the hair prior to cutting

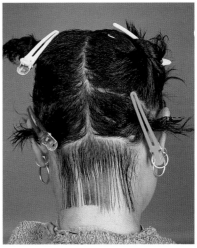

(c) The first section of the guideline cut

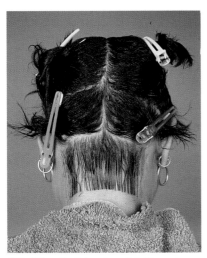

(d) The finished guideline

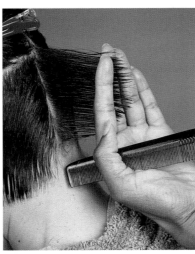

(e) Vertical section held at a 90° angle

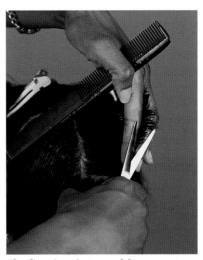

(f) Cutting internal layers at a 90° angle

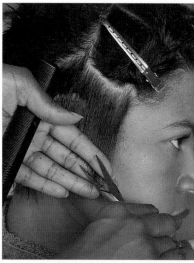

(g) Cutting the side guideline at a 45° angle

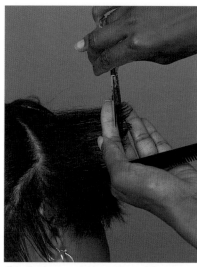

(h) Layer cutting the sides at a 90° angle

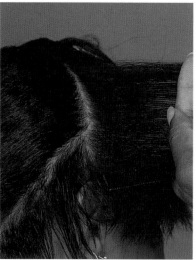

(i) Continuing to cut the sides

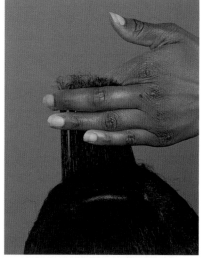

(j) Cutting the horseshoe section at a 90° angle

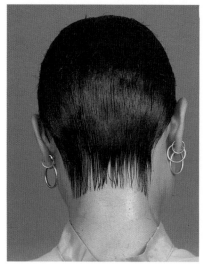

The finished wet cut – back

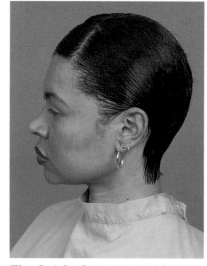

The finished wet cut – side

The finished layered cut after
blow-drying and tonging

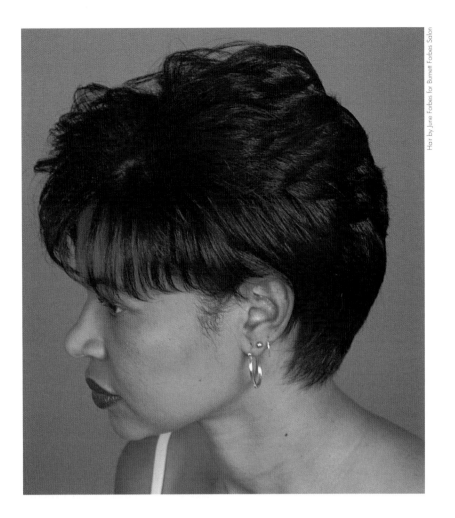

Hair by June Forbes for Burnett Forbes Salon

Long layered/over-directed cut

This cut produces long layers with weight maintained on
the perimeter of the hair, graduating to shorter lengths
internally. It is ideal for clients who want to keep length
but would like movement in a hairstyle or a shorter crown
and fringe area. The internal layers are cut at a 180° angle.

Procedure for long layered cut

1 Follow steps 1 to 3 for an inverted bob on page 160.
2 Divide the hair into four sections and sub-divide into 6
  mm ($\frac{1}{4}$ inch) sub-sections. Cut the hair horizontally on
  the perimeter at a 45° angle (a).
3 Once the guideline has been established, continue to
  bring sections down until you reach the crown (b).
4 Continue the same technique on the sides, blending in
  the back section (c) & (d).

5   Take a horizontal section on the crown and establish the internal guideline. Use this technique to cut the whole horseshoe section until you reach the front hairline (e).

6   Cut the fringe area so it blends with the sides (f) & (g).

7   Starting at the back, blend the internal sections to the crown by taking pie-shaped sections from the crown to the nape (h). Over-direct the hair at a 180° angle and blend the two sections together.

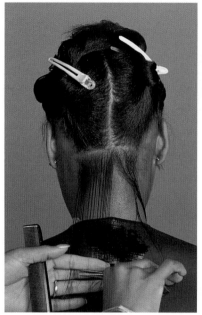

(a) Cutting the guideline at a 45° angle

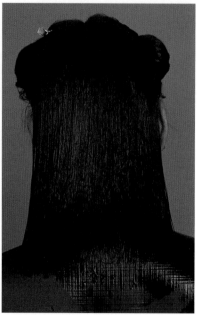

(b) The back after cutting

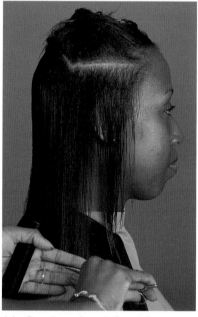

(c) Cutting the right side

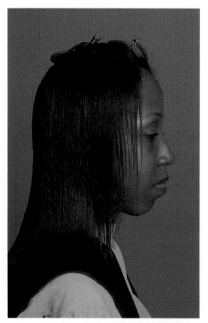

(d) The right side after cutting

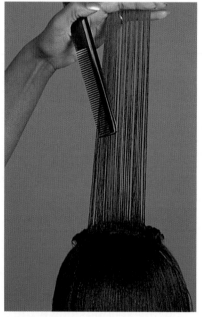

(e) Cutting a horizontal section to establish an internal guideline

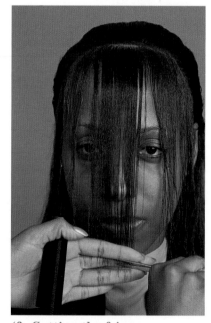

(f) Cutting the fringe

8   Pivot around the head using pie-shaped sections until the crown area is cut.

Note: the hair on the perimeter will not be cut when you use this technique as it will be too short to over-direct to the crown.

9   Cross check the finished cut in the opposite direction (see step 10 for layered cut).

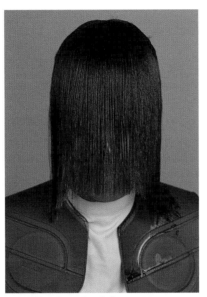

(g) The finished fringe area after cutting

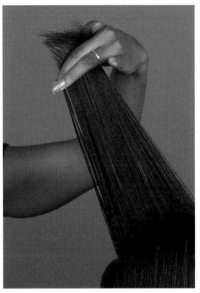

(h) Cutting a pie-shaped section at a 180° angle

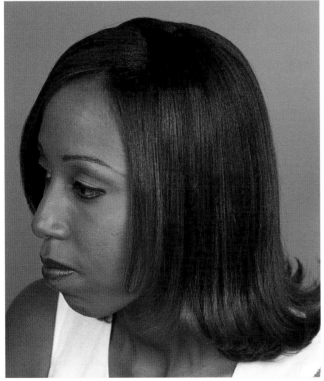

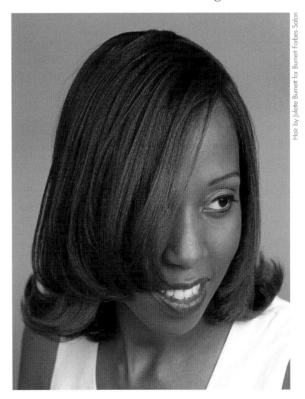

The finished cut after blow-drying and tonging

Fashion cut

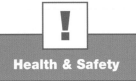
This cut is a combination of more than one cutting technique, used to create a fashion look. Through careful planning and design, a variety of fashion looks can be achieved. It is important to remember that you must have a good understanding of the basics of hair cutting before attempting a fashion cut.

Procedure for fashion cut

1 Follow steps 1 to 3 for an inverted bob on page 160.

2 Start cutting the nape area first. Place the comb under the hair and move the comb in an upwards direction through the hair, with the scissors following the comb, cutting the hair simultaneously. Continue the scissors-over-comb technique up to the occipital bone (a).

3 When the scissors-over-comb technique is completed in the nape area, take a vertical section, hold the hair at a 90° angle and cut. Layer cutting the hair will blend the scissors-over-comb technique and build up weight and length throughout the internal area of the cut (b).

4 Cut the side guideline close to the skin. Once the outline shape has been established, start the scissors-over-comb technique, remembering to blend the back to the sides. Use the same technique to complete the other side (c).

5 Cut the crown area by taking vertical or horizontal sections until you reach the front hairline (d).

6 Take a semicircular guideline, no thicker than 6 mm (0.25 inch). Hold the hair over the forehead using minimum tension and cut the fringe. Bring all the hair

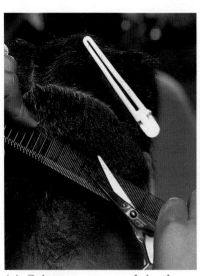

(a) Scissors-over-comb in the nape area

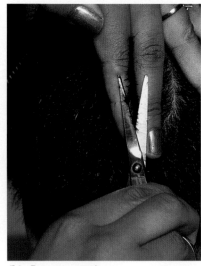

(b) Layer cutting

forward and cut until you run out of hair. Blend the fringe into the sides.

7 Start point-cutting the ends to remove blunt solid ends and create texture within the cut (e).

8 Twist-texturise the fringe and crown to remove weight and add texture to the fringe and crown areas (f) & (g).

9 Cross check the finished cut for balance and shape.

(c) Scissors-over-comb on the sides

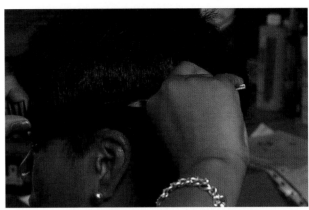

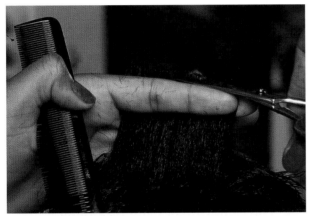

(d) Cutting the crown

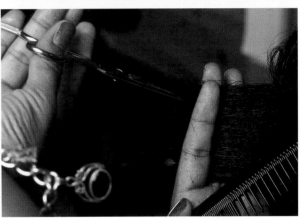

(e) Point-cutting

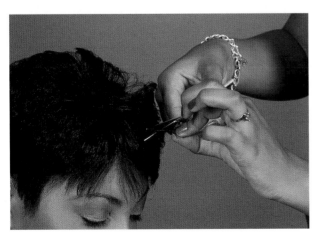

(f) Twist-texturising the fringe

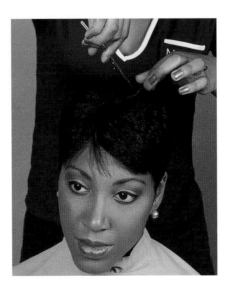

(g) Texturising the crown

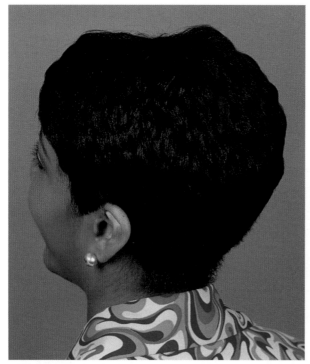

The finished cut – back

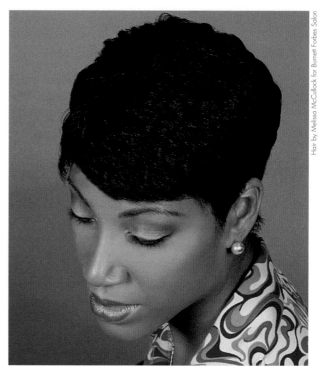

The finished cut – front

Hair by Melissa McCulloch for Burnett Forbes Salon

Sculpture cut

Sculpture cutting is a technique that follows the contours of the head. This technique can be used to create either short or long styles. The sculpture cutting technique was used in the 1960s and 1970s when the Afro hair style was very popular. It allowed the stylist to create a variety of shapes such as round, oval, oblong, square and asymmetric. The technique has always been used for cutting men's hair.

Scissors or **clippers** can be used to achieve the finished look.

- Scissors are used to layer-cut the hair between the fingers. This technique is particularly suitable on texturised or wavy hair which is worn short.
- Clippers are good for cropped looks where a more defined look is required. The stylist can select a variety of attachments which can cut the hair shorter or longer.

Procedure for sculpture cut using scissors

1   Shampoo and condition the hair; comb thoroughly.
2   Take channels, working horizontally through the hair from the nape to the occipital bone. Follow the contours of the head.
3   Blend from the occipital bone to the top of the crown using the same technique as before.
4   Proceed to the sides, taking horizontal sections and using the back as a guideline. Continue cutting until you reach the front hairline. Cut the other side of the hair using the same technique as before.
5   Take vertical or horizontal sections, working from the top of the crown to the front hairline.
6   Cross check the whole cut to make sure it is even.

Procedure for sculpture cut using clippers

1   Shampoo and condition the hair; comb the hair thoroughly and rough dry using the blow-dryer.
2   Comb the hair using an Afro or cutting comb.
3   Keep combing the hair as you proceed through the cut. This will ensure the cut is even and balanced and the required shape is achieved.
4   Select a suitable attachment for the clippers. Start clipper-cutting the hair from the nape. Proceed to the left and then the right side of the head, taking off excess weight and length (a) & (b).

Tip

An aerosol sterilising spray should be used on clippers after use to avoid cross-infection.

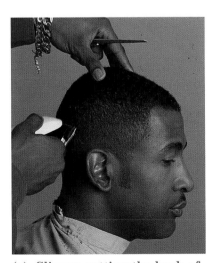

(a) **Clipper-cutting the back of the head**

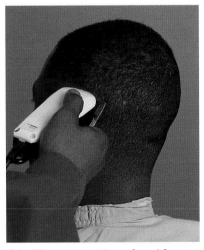

(b) **Clipper-cutting the sides**

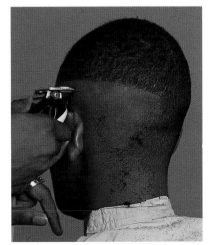

(c) **Marking out areas to be faded**

5   Mark out the area to be faded, working from the nape up to the temple (c).

6   Cut the hair on the crown in channels, starting in the middle. Once the desired length has been established, cut the rest of the crown (d).

7   Blend the faded area to the crown, working in channels until you reach the front hairline (e) & (f).

8   Cross check by combing the hair after the initial cut. Remove any uneven hair with the clippers.

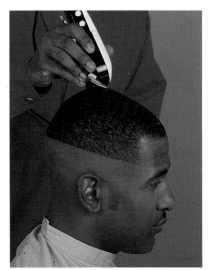

(d) Cutting the crown

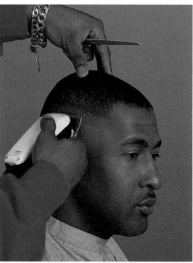

(e) Blending the faded area to the crown

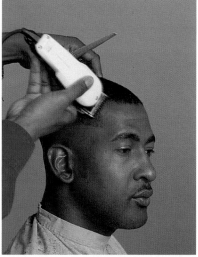

(f) Cutting the hair in channels

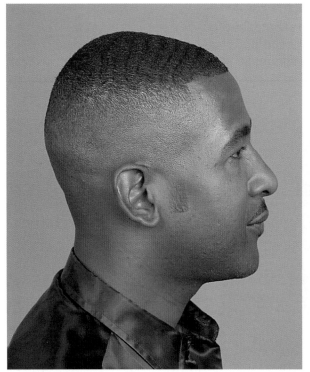

The finished cut – side

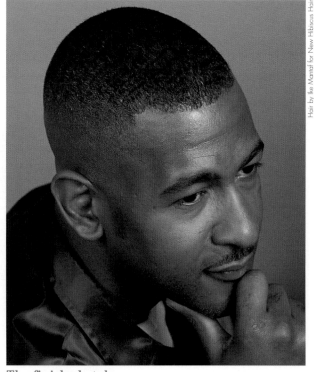

The finished style

Hair by Ike Mantof for New Hibiscus Hair

Colouring

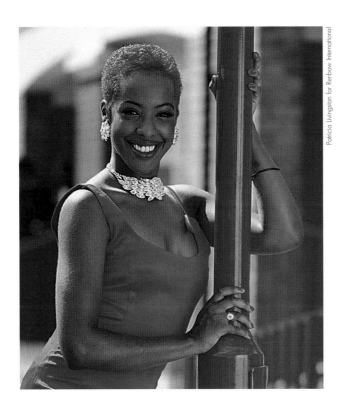

Patricia Livingston for Renbow International

11

Learning objectives

This chapter covers the following:

- **the science of colouring**

- **consultation and analysis**

- **different types of colouring processes**

- **bleaching**

- **fashion techniques**

- **colour correction and restoration**

- **reduction of colourants**

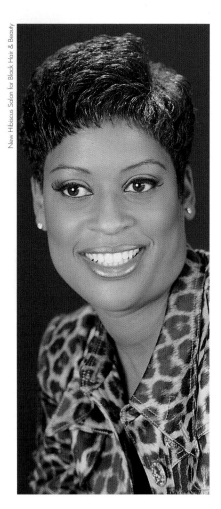

New Hibiscus Salon for Black Hair & Beauty

The desire to change one's natural hair colour in favour of another is not a new concept. As long as 2000 years ago, the Africans and Egyptians were making use of the henna plant to add variety to their hair colour. Henna, although still favoured by some, has given way to more cosmetically designed means of colouring the hair. Today, hair colouring is achieved by the addition to the hair of one or several pigments in the form of synthetic dyes, or by the removal of the natural pigment from the hair.

These colourants range from:

- **temporary**, which lasts for only one shampoo
- **semi-permanent**, which lasts for 6–8 shampoos
- **quasi-permanent** which lasts for 8–12 shampoos
- **permanent**, which cannot be shampooed out of the hair but will disappear as the hair is cut over a period of time
- **vegetable**, which can behave like permanent colourants in that they produce a line of regrowth.

In the past there has been a reluctance by both stylists and clients alike to venture into the area of permanently colouring African-Caribbean hair due to its delicate nature, especially when working with hair which has been previously processed with either a relaxer or permanent wave product. However, improved products and technology have given rise to exciting colour options for African-Caribbean clients, provided all necessary precautions are taken as discussed later in the chapter.

Why colour?

Colouring hair allows the client freedom of expression and maintains individuality. For the stylist, it expands imagination and creative ability, allowing you to dramatise a haircut by adding colour in strategic places, to make an old hairstyle more interesting or simply to allow you to offer an additional service to the client.

The science of colouring

What is colour?

Colour is an optical illusion – a reflection of light falling onto the object in view. In hair, the outer layer (the cuticle) is translucent and it is the colour pigments in the cortex which shine through the cuticle and give us the colour that we see on the hair.

Colour composition

Synthetic colour is made up from the three primary pigment colours: red, yellow and blue. When two primary colours are mixed together, they produce secondary colours: orange, green or violet, and form the basis for synthetic hair-colouring products.

Natural hair colour

All natural hair consists of varying proportions of black, brown, red and yellow pigments. Black and brown hair contains a lot of pigment, mostly the very dark pigment, **eumelanin**. Blonde hair contains very little pigment, predominantly the yellow-red pigment **pheomelanin**. White hair has very little or no melanin. This loss of pigment occurs naturally as part of the ageing process. However, you may come across a person whose hair has very little or no pigment, with pigment also lacking from the eyes and skin. This is known as albinism or semi-albinism.

Grey hair tends to be a mixture of white and coloured hairs. Depending on the tone of the hair, it is possible to identify which pigments are present, for example if the hair is reddish brown then there will also be some red pigments, notably **trichosiderin**.

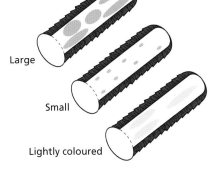

Large

Small

Lightly coloured

Types of pigment granules

The difference in African-Caribbean hair

Pigment is mainly found in the cortex of the hair. However, some Oriental and African-Caribbean hair types also have pigment distributed in the cuticle. Research suggests that African-Caribbean hair is more resistant to the penetration of chemicals. This, however, is only true for hair in its virgin state. Once the hair has been chemically processed with either a relaxer or permanent wave product, the hair becomes more porous and absorption of any colouring agent takes place quickly (see Chapter 2).

In African-Caribbean hair, the pigment granules are larger than in other hair types and they appear less frequently. This allows them to be broken down quickly when using oxidation tints. When certain colouring services are carried out, such as tinting and bleaching, the arrangement of the natural pigments is altered to embrace the introduction of the new colour pigments.

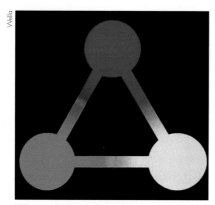

The colour triangle

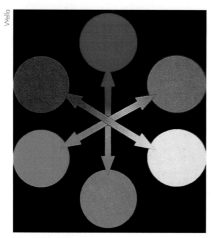

The colour circle

How is colour made up?

When colouring hair, pigments are used in a similar way to paints. They can either be used separately or mixed together to achieve different colours. There are four main sets of colours: primary, secondary, tertiary and complementary.

Primary colours: red, yellow and blue

These colours cannot be created by mixing pigments together. However, when all three primary colours are mixed together in varying quantities, shades ranging from black to very light brown can be obtained.

Secondary colours: orange, green and violet

These are obtained when two primary colours are mixed together:

- red + yellow = orange
- yellow + blue = green
- blue + red = violet.

Tertiary colours

These are obtained when equal proportions of adjacent primary and secondary colours are mixed together (see illustration of colour circle). These give the more vibrant fashion shades and can also be used for corrective colouring (see page 212).

- red + orange = copper red (chestnut)
- orange + yellow = gold
- yellow + green = lime green (seen in fashion colours)
- green + blue = ash
- blue + violet = pearl
- violet + red = mahogany.

Red, orange and yellow are known as warm colours; green, blue and violet are known as cool colours.

Complementary colours

Complementary colours are made up of a primary and a secondary colour which are opposite each other on the colour star. They can be used to neutralise unwanted hair colour and, when mixed together, produce a shade of brown.

Neutralising unwanted hair colour

'Neutralising' colour is a way of getting rid of unwanted colour which has emerged during the tinting process. Any colour can be neutralised by the addition of its opposite colour in the colour circle (see table).

Unwanted hair colour	Corrective colour
Too much yellow	Cool violet (mauve)
Too much orange	Cool blue (ash)
Green	Red
Violet	Yellow (golds)
Blue	Orange (coppers)

Depth and tone

Depth is how dark or light a colour is, depending on the proportion of pigments in the hair. With artificial colours, if more black is used then the colour will be darker. If more white is used, then the colour will be lighter. **Tone** is the colour we actually see, therefore brown will be the depth of the colour whereas reddish brown would indicate a red tone.

Consultation and analysis

Shade charts

To simplify the colouring procedure, manufacturers produce shade charts using synthetic hair swatches in order to show their colour range. It is important when choosing a colour for the client, to ascertain the client's natural depth by holding the hair swatch as close to the root of the hair as possible. Then make sure that the client looks at the target colour in natural light as salon lighting can often distort colour.

All shade charts have to conform to the **International Colour Chart System (ICC)**, showing a numbering system to differentiate between the different colours. These are numbered from 1–10 or, for some companies, from 1–11. Some companies also employ a number and letter system

Stylist and client selecting a
suitable colour

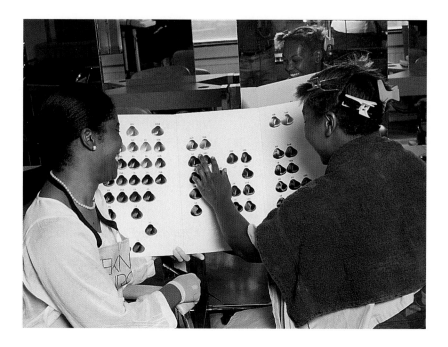

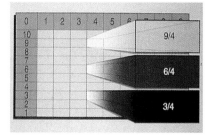

Depths and tones

along with the colour identification name. The numbers and
letters will tell you, the hairdresser, what depth and tone
the colour is. However, not all manufacturers apply the
same numbering system to the various colours.

Most shade charts will include a selection of concentrated
colours which can be used with the other colours in the
range to produce more vibrant tones. Therefore, if a client
would like a red-brown colour but wants the red to be
vibrant, you can add a measured amount of concentrated
red to achieve more vibrancy.

Due to the fact that African-Caribbean hair is usually dark
in colour, it is often impossible to achieve some of the
lighter colours without pre-lightening the hair. Shade
charts can be used very effectively to assist you in showing
the client the colour that is achievable with and without
pre-lightening. However, it is necessary to bear in mind the
number of lifts required to achieve the desired colour, the
volume of hydrogen peroxide to be used, the chemicals
already on the hair and the information gathered from an
analysis of the hair before making a final decision as to the
target colour.

Recording information

It is important to have a separate record card, giving a
brief outline of your findings from your tests and analysis
of the hair. This will enable another stylist to carry
out subsequent colouring services if you are
unavailable.

Tip

All information gathered
must be recorded on a
client record card.

COLOUR RECORD CARD

Client's name .... Address ....

....

Tel .... Natural hair colour ....

Percentage of white hair ....

Date	Stylist	Type	Full head/ Regrowth	Target colour	Preparation method	Hydrogen peroxide	Comment

Colour analysis sheet

Name:

Address:

Tel:

Date:

1 What type of colouring process does the client require? ....

   Temporary ☐ semi-permanent ☐ quasi-permanent ☐ permanent ☐ bleaching ☐

2 Has the client had a skin test? Yes ☐ No ☐ Date of test: ....

3 Does the scalp reveal any conditions which will prohibit the colouring process (abrasions, cuts, infections)?

   ....

4 Texture: Fine   ☐   Medium ☐   Coarse   ☐

5 Porosity   Porous ☐   Normal ☐   Resistant ☐

6 Has the client had any other chemical services: Yes ☐   No ☐   Relaxer ☐   Permanent wave ☐

7 Incompatability test   Yes ☐ No ☐

8 Elasticity test: Good ☐ Average ☐ Poor ☐

9 Full head ☐ or regrowth application ☐

10 Has a test cutting been carried out? If so, what was used and the result achieved

   ....

11 Strand test (see notes below) ....

12 What is the client's natural base shade?

13 Target colour: ....

14 Shade of previous colour (if any) ....

15 Percentage and distribution of white hair: .... Is it resistant white hair? Yes ☐ No ☐

16 Colour developer/peroxide strength to be used:

17 Processing time allowed on the roots/ends:

18 Result achieved/comments:

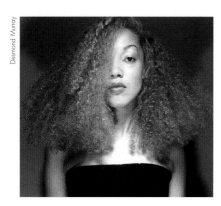

Notes on carrying out analysis

For colouring options see page 189.

1   It is important to carry out a skin test before any colouring process involving the use of 'para' dyes (see below).

2   Be sure to note any irritation to the scalp. This might have been caused by sensitisation from relaxers or perms which may leave the scalp tender. If there is any evidence of irritation, do not proceed with colouring service but allow scalp to heal.

3   The texture of the hair will affect the development time as coarse hair may be more resistant than fine hair. It is important to remember, however, that all hair textures, whether coarse, medium or fine, will absorb colour more quickly once relaxed or permanent-waved.

4   Porosity – this will also affect development time as porous hair will absorb colour quickly (see pages 5–6).

5   Other chemicals on the hair will automatically make the hair slightly porous.

6   Incompatability test – this tests for metallic substances which may be present in the hair due to the use of colour restorers. These react with hydrogen peroxide and can cause breakage (see pages 185–6).

7   Elasticity test – this checks the condition of the hair to see whether it is strong enough to accept a(nother) chemical (see page 5).

8   Full head or regrowth application will determine your method of application, either roots first or mid-lengths, ends and then roots.

9   Test-cutting – this is carried out before the colouring or bleaching service and will determine the development time and whether the chosen colour is achievable (see page 186).

10 Strand test – this is carried out during the colouring service and checks the colour development from the roots to ends.

11 The client's natural base shade will give an indication of the underlying predominant pigment and whether you will need to use a complementary colour instead of the target colour to neutralise any unwanted colour which may emerge.

12 Target colour – is it lighter or darker than the natural base shade? This will determine the strength of peroxide to use (if necessary).

13 Shade of previous colour (if any) – this will be seen on the mid-lengths to ends of hair. Check for colour fade and whether you need to refresh colour on the ends.

The above tests will reveal the colouring options available to your client.

Skin tests

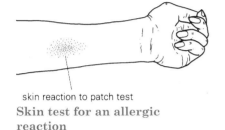

skin reaction to patch test

Skin test for an allergic reaction

It is necessary to carry out a skin test before using colouring products which contain para-phenylenediamine or para-toluenediamine, otherwise known as 'para' dyes. These dyes will either be permanent or quasi-permanent and will be identified as such on any packaging. Skin tests check for any allergic reactions to 'para' and are usually carried out 24–48 hours before colour application.

Procedure

1 Protect the client with a gown and towel.
2 Mix peroxide and tint, using the same volume peroxide that you intend to use on the client.
3 Clean either the inside of the elbow or behind the ear with surgical spirit and cotton wool.
4 Apply a small amount of tint to the area and leave to dry.
5 Ask the client to leave the skin test for 24–48 hours. If the skin test gives a negative result, it is possible to go ahead with the colouring service. If, however, an allergic reaction occurs, the area will become red, sore, begin to itch or swell. The client must be advised to wash the area immediately and notify the salon of any positive reaction. If the irritation persists, advise the client to seek medical attention.
6 Record the result on the client's record card (see sample record card on page 183).

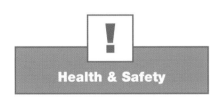

Health & Safety

Do not apply tint to a client who has had a positive reaction to a skin test. Other colouring services should be offered, such as highlights (preferably cap highlights), temporary colours, vegetable colours and some semi-permanents, making sure that the latter do not contain 'para' dyes. It is also important to stress to clients the gravity of the consequences should they then decide to shop around for another hairdresser who will carry out a colouring service using 'para' dyes.

Incompatibility test

This tests for the presence of metallic salts on the hair. Metallic salts are generally found in hair colour restorers, some coloured hairsprays and compound vegetable dyes. They are incompatible with any product requiring the use of hydrogen peroxide.

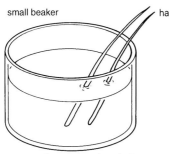

small beaker / hair

no reaction – hair and product
are compatible

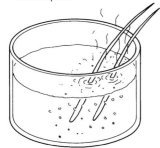

reaction (between chemicals
in lotion and chemicals already
on hair) – hair and product
lotion are incompatible

Incompatibility test

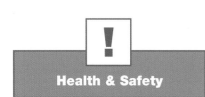

Health & Safety

Do not apply products which
require the use of hydrogen
peroxide to hair which has
shown a positive
incompatibility reading as this
could result in breakage and
chemical burns to the skin.
Again, stress to the client the
consequences of not taking note
of the result of the test. If
necessary, show them the test
and advise them not to try to
get the service carried out
elsewhere.

Procedure

1   Use protective gloves.
2   Take a sample of hair and place it in a mixture of
    hydrogen peroxide and ammonium hydroxide. If
    heating, discoloration or bubbling takes place, this
    suggests that there are incompatible chemicals present
    on the hair.

Test cutting

So far so good! The next stage is to carry out a test cutting
to ensure that the chosen colour is achievable and to
ascertain the approximate length of time it will take for the
colour to develop.

Procedure

1   Cut a small amount of hair, preferably from the back of
    the head where the hair is thickest, and secure it with
    thread or sellotape.
2   Mix the chosen colour with the appropriate strength
    peroxide and apply to a hair sample.
3   Leave to develop, allowing extra time for development
    due to lack of body heat.
4   Check the result and compare it with the target
    colour.

Strand test

This is carried out *during* the colour service and checks the
colour development from the roots to the ends.

Procedure

1   Follow the manufacturer's instructions regarding
    processing time.
2   Using a damp piece of cotton wool, remove tint from a
    strand of hair so as to assess the colour.
3   Make sure that it is an even colour from roots to
    ends.
4   Remove the tint if the colour is even. If it is not even,
    leave to process for a further length of time or apply
    more tint if necessary.

Hydrogen peroxide

Hydrogen peroxide is the active ingredient which is used as a catalyst to activate tints and bleaches by providing oxygen. In its chemical structure, it is similar to that of water, except that hydrogen peroxide has an extra oxygen atom attached to it.

Water = H_2O Hydrogen Peroxide = H_2O_2

During the chemical process of tinting or bleaching, oxygen is given off due to the interaction of ammonia which is found in tints, bleach and hydrogen peroxide. Hydrogen peroxide is therefore called an oxidising agent.

Hydrogen peroxide comes in different strengths which can be measured in percentage strength (%) or volume strength (vol.). Percentage strength tells us how many parts of pure hydrogen peroxide are found in 100 parts of pure solution. Therefore a 6% solution would contain 6 grams of pure hydrogen peroxide in 100 grams of solution.

Volume strength is the number of parts of free oxygen that one part of hydrogen peroxide would give off during the oxidation process. Therefore 1 ml of 20 vol. hydrogen peroxide gives 20 ml free oxygen.

The stronger the hydrogen peroxide, the more oxygen is given off. Therefore 1 litre of 20 vol. would give off 20 litres of oxygen, whilst 1 litre of 40 vol. would give off 40 litres of oxygen. Due to the fact that it is the oxygen which is given off from the hydrogen peroxide that brings about the oxidation process, the higher the level of hydrogen peroxide, the stronger the result.

When working with hydrogen peroxide it is wise to note that the product is at its most effective immediately after mixing. This is particularly important when working with full head applications of tints/bleach or highlights/lowlights. If mixed tint or bleach is still in use after half an hour of mixing, the product will work more slowly as it will have oxidised too much. It is better to mix fresh product for a more even result.

Different strengths of hydrogen peroxide are used as follows:

- 10 vol. or 3% – used for toning, e.g. bleach toners
- 20 vol. or 6% – used to deposit colour when tinting, i.e. white coverage, or can be used to lighten base shade by 1 lift.
- 30 vol. or 9% – used to lighten base shade by up to 2 lifts
- 40 vol. or 12% – used mainly for highlighting and will lighten base shade by 3 lifts.

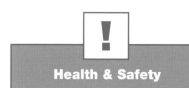

Health & Safety

The darker the base shade of the client, the higher the strength of hydrogen peroxide you would need to use to achieve the lighter colours. Whilst it is possible to use the full range of hydrogen peroxide strengths on African-Caribbean hair, care must be taken especially when another chemical is already on the hair, such as a relaxer or perm or, in the case of virgin hair, if the client intends to have an additional chemical service to the hair at some stage. It is advisable to carry out an incompatibility test (page 185) along with a strand test (page 186).

White hair coverage

When using quasi-permanent or permanent colours it is important to note whether the client has any grey hair present. In order to cover grey, additional colour of a natural shade in the same target number of your target colour will need to be applied. For example, if there is grey hair present and your target shade is 7K (copper) then you need to add a percentage of 7N (N for the natural shade) to the 7K in order to cover the white hair.

Very often, stylists become confused with which of the natural shades to add to the tint. Do not add the client's natural base shade because this will make the overall colour too dark or have the effect of not covering the white areas adequately, depending on whether you are going from a dark colour to a light colour or vice versa.

Use the table below to help you to decide how much of the natural shade to include.

% of white	Natural tone needed (in millilitres)	Target tone needed (in millilitres)
10–30%	15 ml	25 ml
40–60%	20 ml	20 ml
70–100%	25 ml	15 ml

Most manufacturers recommend that tints be mixed equal part hydrogen peroxide to equal part tint. Therefore, for a full head application, depending on length, a mixture of 40 ml of hydrogen peroxide of the desired strength and 40 ml of the target shade should be mixed together. However, if white hair is present, the mixture is different as some natural tone needs to be added. Using the table above, if the client is a base of 4N with 40% white hair and requires a target shade of 6B (brown) then it is necessary to add 20 ml of natural tone which is 6N, plus 20 ml of the target tone which is 6B. Together this makes a total of 40 ml of tint which should be added to 40 ml of 30 vol. (2 levels of lift) for a full head application (see page 187 for peroxide strengths).

Resistant hair

You will come across hair which is resistant to tint. This is generally hair which is coated with products or hair which has a tightly packed cuticle so that penetration of chemicals does not take place easily. White hair sometimes falls into this category. However, it is important to note that white hair can 'grab' certain colours such as reds more easily than others.

Tip

If the hair has been styled with heavy oils or gels, it will be resistant to tint because the oils/gels act as a barrier. It will therefore be necessary to gently shampoo the hair first before proceeding with the tinting process. Dry hair under a cool dryer to avoid sensitising the scalp.

When using dark colours, tint the white hair first, especially around the hairline. When working with lighter colours tint the white hair last.

Choosing a colour

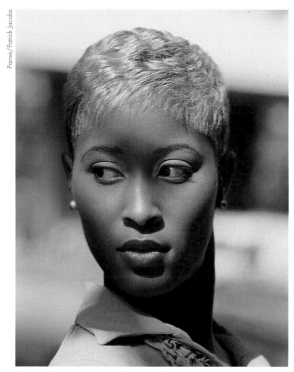

Hair bleached and toned

We are now ready to start our tinting service. There are many colours to choose from. It is wise, before you show the client the shade chart, to discuss what colour she has in mind. This will help you to pick out about three or four colours from which the client could choose. It is better to look at these colours in natural daylight by the window or even outside as salon lighting may distort colour.

At this stage you can take into consideration the client's age, job, mode of dress, lifestyle, skin tone and the results from your analysis of the hair, to help you to narrow your options down to one or two colours. Remember that your colour options may be reduced by the presence of other chemicals such as a relaxer or permanent wave.

Very often a client may try to persuade you to carry out a colouring service which you think may endanger the hair. Remember always to rely on the results of your tests and analysis. Be gentle but firm if you believe that the result could be problematic – your reputation is at stake.

Colouring options

Different colouring options are available to your client. These can be classified under four headings: temporary, semi-permanent, quasi-permanent and permanent. They are identified by their life span on the hair.

- **temporary** – lasts for one shampoo
- **semi-permanent** – lasts through 6 to 8 shampoos
- **quasi-permanent** – lasts through 8 to 12 shampoos and may contain 'para' (see page 185). Could last longer on porous hair and may even produce a line of regrowth.
- **permanent** – does not shampoo out but grows out as new hair emerges. Contains 'para' (see page 185).

Colourants are derived from a variety of sources such as vegetable, vegetable and mineral, and mineral.

Vegetable colourants

Vegetable colourants have been in use for centuries, mainly in the Middle East and Northern Africa. In the 1980s vegetable colourants were very popular with African-Caribbean clients as this was a means of colouring the hair with minimum damage. Previous to this, some had experimented with permanent hair colouring products which were primarily for Caucasian use. Whilst there was nothing wrong with that, they were unable to achieve the lighter hair colours due to the predominant underlying red pigment, trichosiderin, found in African-Caribbean hair. The only other option was to bleach the hair which, if not carried out with care, could irreparably damage the hair. Thereafter colouring African-Caribbean hair was viewed with some scepticism and thenceforth vegetable-based colouring products became very popular albeit limiting in the choice of colours which were available.

However, some vegetable colourants posed problems in that when they were used on hair which was not chemically treated with either a relaxer or permanent wave they performed well, but when chemicals were already on the hair they sometimes rendered the hair unsuitable for subsequent chemical services. This was due to the fact that a vegetable colourant such as henna would attach itself to the cystine bonds in the hair causing uneven absorption. This, coupled with the fact that relaxers and permanent wave chemicals were not as sophisticated as they are now, meant that damage often occurred.

In the final analysis, it is wise to rely on the results of your analysis and tests before deciding whether to go ahead with any vegetable colouring service.

The main vegetable colourants are camomile and henna.

Camomile

Camomile is usually added to shampoos and conditioners and is used to achieve yellow/gold tones. Due to the fact that African-Caribbean hair is dark in colour, camomile-based products are only of benefit if the hair has been pre-lightened. Even then it would only serve to enhance pre-lightened areas.

Henna

Henna is probably the most widely known vegetable colourant. It is derived from the henna bush (*Lawsonia alba*) and is especially known and used for its conditioning

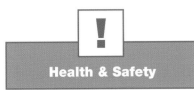

Health & Safety

Henna should not be confused with compound henna, which is henna combined with minerals or metallic salts. This was used to widen the range of colours from henna. Such compound hennas react violently with hydrogen peroxide – an incompatability test will reveal whether metallic salts are present (see page 185).

Tip

When using henna that contains an additional substance such as metallic salts, a skin test should be carried out prior to use, as this type of product can cause an allergic reaction.

properties. Although henna can lose some of its colour on shampooing, it can be classified as a permanent colour because it results in the need for regrowth application. This is due to the fact that henna is a natural oxidation dye – the colour develops gradually as the dye molecules are slowly oxidised by the oxygen in the air. Over several applications the properties in henna can attach to the protein (keratin) in hair and therefore create a build-up.

Henna is able to deposit in both the cuticle and the cortex layers but, unlike permanent colour, it does not cover grey hair and cannot lighten hair. There is no need to carry out a skin test prior to application. It does, however, have the benefit of sealing the cuticle which gives the hair a high sheen. Henna is naturally red in colour. However, additional powdered substances are often added to henna to make up other shades, for example the addition of indigo leaves results in a blue-black colour.

Application method

1   Choose a henna shade and put the required amount into a large enough bowl for mixing (see manufacturer's instructions).

2   Add sufficient boiling water from a boiled kettle to mix the henna into a smooth paste.

3   Leave the paste to cool.

4   Gown and towel the client.

5   Apply a barrier cream to the client's hairline and section the hair into four.

6   Check the henna mix to ensure that it has cooled down sufficiently to be applied to the hair.

7   Put on gloves and using a brush, apply henna from roots to ends, starting at the nape area first. Take larger sections than you would for applying a tint (page 198).

8   Put a strip of cotton wool around the hairline and cover the head with a plastic cap.

9   Place the client under a preheated dryer for about 15–30 minutes or more depending on the depth of colour you require (1 hour is usually more than adequate).

10   Once processing time is over, rinse the hair thoroughly using warm water until all the mixture is out of the hair. Shampoo the hair, preferably with an acid balanced shampoo. Towel dry and style accordingly.

Vegetable and mineral colourants

These are a combination of vegetable and mineral substances such as the compound henna mentioned above.

Mineral colourants

These fall into two categories:

- **Metallic dyes** are mainly found in hair restorers and only coat the surface of the hair.
- **Aniline derivatives** are synthetic dyes made from substances found in crude oil.

Whilst aniline derivitives fall under the category of mineral colourants, they operate very differently from the inorganic metallic dyes. Aniline derivative are used in semi-permanent, quasi-permanent and permanent colourants and are commonly known as 'para' dyes. They can be used simply to tint the hair or to lighten the natural hair colour and deposit a tint simultaneously.

Temporary colourants

Temporary colourants are exactly as the name suggests – they only colour the hair temporarily. This is because the colour molecules in temporary colourants are so large that they cannot penetrate the hair shaft unless the hair is excessively porous. The colour molecules only coat the surface of the hair and last only one shampoo. Temporary colourants can be applied without a skin test.

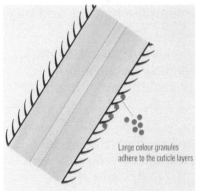

Large colour granules adhere to the cuticle layers

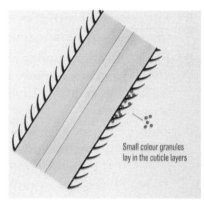

Small colour granules lay in the cuticle layers

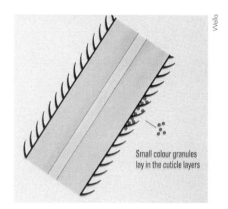

Small colour granules lay in the cuticle layers

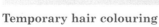

Temporary hair colouring

Types of temporary colours

- **setting lotions** – coloured plastic setting lotions and blow-dry lotions
- **gels or foams** – coloured mousses and gels
- **water rinses** – concentrated colour drops added to very hot water
- **coloured hairsprays** – these may contain metallic particles of gold and silver which in the past were often dyed aluminium particles
- **crayons/hair mascaras** – these are mainly used around the hairline or in small areas where colour is required. The crayon is lightly stroked against the area to be coloured.

Temporary colours can be used:

- to enhance dull looking hair – temporary colour will not lighten hair but will revitalise natural colour.
- to blend white hair
- to get rid of a yellowish tinge in grey hair
- to add colour to hair which has been pre-lightened.

Unless the hair has been pre-lightened, only certain temporary colours will be effective on African-Caribbean hair. Colours such as blue-black, brown, red, burgundy and copper will add more depth/warmth to the client's natural colour.

Application

Most temporary colour products do not require mixing and can therefore be used straight from the container.

1 Gown and protect the client with a suitable towel for colouring.
2 Wear rubber gloves as staining of the hands may occur.
3 Avoid the colour touching the scalp and hairline as staining will occur.
4 Care must be taken to apply colour evenly.

- **Water rinses:** hair must be shampooed prior to applying coloured water rinse. The water rinse will be the final rinse. Hair is then towel dried and styled as required.

Health & Safety

Hairsprays containing metallic particles may cause breakage or interference with chemical processes.

Tip

The use of coloured setting lotions and mousses which are not specifically designed for African-Caribbean hair could temporarily make the hair dry due to their alcohol content.

- **Coloured setting lotions and mousses:** hair must be shampooed and towel dried before applying. Too much water left in the hair will dilute the effect of the setting lotion/mousse. They can be applied by hand or using a comb to run through the hair thereby giving even coverage.

- **Coloured hairsprays:** these are applied to dry hair. Care must be taken to protect clothes, skin and areas of the hair which do not require colouring. If too much hairspray is applied to the hair, it will have to be shampooed out and the hair restyled.

Remember to check coloured hairsprays to see if they contain metallic particles. If they do, it is wise not to use on hair which is already chemically processed with either a relaxer or permanent wave product as there will be incompatibility of products (see Chapters 7 and 8 for more information).

Semi-permanent colourants

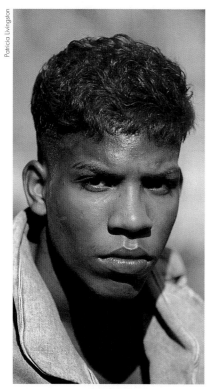

Patricia Livingston

Pre-lightened hair toned with blue semi-permanent colour

Semi-permanent colourants are different from temporary colourants in that the colour molecules are smaller and are therefore able to partly penetrate to the outer cortex of the hair. It therefore takes about six to eight shampoos before a semi-permanent colourant is washed out of the hair completely. Retouching is not necessary because the colour fades away naturally without leaving a line of regrowth. Should the client wish to retain the same colour then it will be necessary to carry out a full head application again.

Types of semi-permanent colourant

Semi-permanent colourants consist of mixtures of nitro-phenylenediamine (red and yellow colours) and anthraquinones (blue colours). However, some also contain paraphenylene-diamine (more commonly known as 'para') found in tints. They come in the form of creams and lotions.

Semi-permanent colourants can be used:

- to enhance dull looking hair
- to add colour to pre-lightened hair
- to blend grey hair.

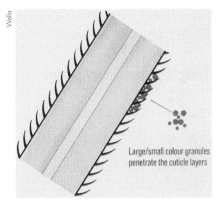

Semi-permanent hair colouring

Tip

Due to the fact that African-Caribbean hair tends to be dark in colour it is not possible to achieve light hair colours with semi-permanents as they do not lighten the hair. Semi-permanents are mainly used on African-Caribbean hair type to enhance the natural colour, to add red and golden highlights, to tone pre-lightened hair and to blend grey hair.

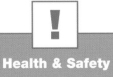

Health & Safety

Semi-permanent colourants do not alter the chemical balance of the hair. However, if the hair is excessively porous, colour will grab more easily and uneven colouring may occur in areas which are more porous than others.

Application

Some semi-permanent colourants can be used straight from the container. Others, which may need to be mixed, should be applied using a tint bowl and tint brush.

1   Gown and protect client using a dark towel and tinting gown.

2   Shampoo the hair prior to application of semi-permanent colourants. This cleanses the hair and opens the cuticle to allow penetration.

3   Towel dry the hair to remove excess water which could dilute the product.

4   Wear rubber gloves to avoid staining of the nails and hands.

5   Ensure that there is sufficient product. One bottle may not be sufficient, especially if the hair is long.

6   Apply product, starting from the nape area where the hair is more resistant, using an applicator bottle, sponge or tinting brush.

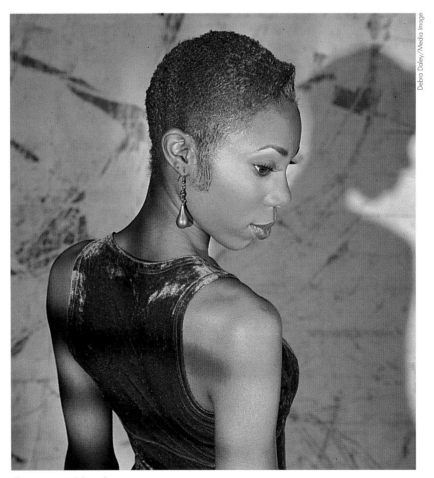

Copper gold colour

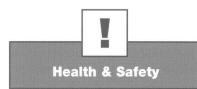

7   Take neat, even partings and work up towards the hairline. Care must be taken to apply colour evenly, working from roots to ends.

8   Avoid the colour touching the scalp and hairline as staining will occur.

9   Cross check application to ensure all the hair is covered. It is always wise to cross check in the opposite direction to which the product was applied.

10 Use a wide-toothed comb to ensure that the colour is applied evenly and to sufficiently loosen the hair to allow air to circulate freely, especially if additional heat is required.

11 Apply cotton strip around the hairline to ensure the colour does not come into contact with any other areas such as the eyes, face, neck and ears.

12 Check the manufacturer's instructions to see if the addition of a plastic cap or drier is required.

13 Allow the colour to develop, following the manufacturer's directions. It can take between 5 and 30 minutes for semi-permanent colourant to enter the cortex.

14 Check development by removing some product from the hair with a damp piece of cotton wool and placing the hair over a fresh piece of cotton wool to get a better reading of the colour achieved.

15 Once development has taken place, rinse the hair thoroughly at the basin until the water runs clear. Do not shampoo the hair at this stage as colour fade will begin to take place.

16 Remove any stains on the skin or scalp with cotton wool and stain remover. Rinse thoroughly and style as desired.

Quasi-permanent colourants

Tip

Some quasi-permanent colours will produce a regrowth on very porous hair, e.g. relaxed or permed hair.

These colourants are not permanent. However, they are generally mixed with a very low volume peroxide. This allows them to enter the cortex where they enlarge and cannot easily be shampooed out of the hair. They last between 8–12 shampoos which is longer than the other non-permanent hair colourants. Quasi-permanent colourants do not lighten natural hair colour because they use only 'low strength' peroxide.

Quasi-permanent colourants can be used:

● to add colour to pre-lightened hair

Health & Safety

Always carry out a skin test before using 'para' dyes. Quasi-permanent colourants contain a small amount of 'para', therefore a skin test is necessary (see page 185).

Tip

Due to the depth of colour of African-Caribbean hair, only certain colours in the quasi-permanent range can be effectively used for colour change. Colours such as reds and blue-black are the most effective, but dark brown can be used in hair which is mid to light brown in colour.

- to tone hair which has been coloured/highlighted
- to refresh old highlights
- to refresh ends of permanently coloured hair when carrying out a regrowth application
- to add gloss to natural hair
- to blend grey hair
- to introduce new colours to clients without the commitment of a permanent colourant.

Permanent hair colouring/oxidation tints

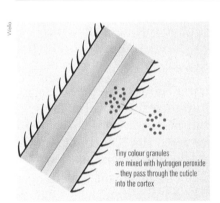

Tiny colour granules are mixed with hydrogen peroxide – they pass through the cuticle into the cortex

Permanent hair colouring is a process whereby the natural pigment in the hair is changed by means of a chemical oxidation process (see page 187). There is quite a wide range of colours to choose from. However, not all of these colours are achievable on African-Caribbean hair due to the depth of the natural hair colour. To achieve the lighter hair colours, bleaching will first have to be carried out.

Although the word **permanent** is used, the process is only permanent in the hair which has been tinted and does not refer to any subsequent regrowth.

Types of permanent colours

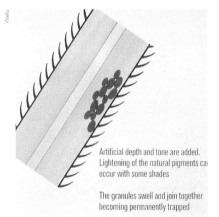

Artificial depth and tone are added. Lightening of the natural pigments can occur with some shades

The granules swell and join together becoming permanently trapped

Permanent hair colouring

Permanent tints come in the form of creams, gels or cream/gel mixtures. They are synthetic in make-up and have to be mixed with hydrogen peroxide for the product to become active. The chemical reaction between the tints and the hydrogen peroxide brings about an oxidation reaction of the hair's natural pigment, thereby removing the natural colour from the hair, while depositing the new colour from the tint into the hair.

When it is freshly mixed, the 'para', which is found in all permanent tints, is colourless and its molecules are small

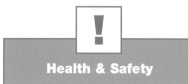

Health & Safety

Always carry out a skin test before using 'para' dyes (see page 185).

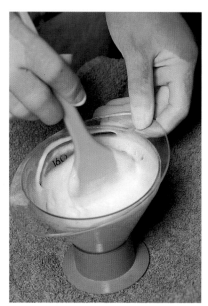

Preparing the tint

Tip

Manufacturers tend to produce a large range of shades of tints. However, they can be intermixed, within the range, to suit individual needs.

enough to penetrate the cortex of the hair. As it oxidises, the small molecules combine to form larger molecules which are then too large to be shampooed out of the hair.

Permanent colourants can be used:

- to darken or to lighten existing hair using either full head application method or regrowth application method
- to add colour tone to existing hair
- to cover white hair
- to neutralise unwanted colour tones
- to highlight, apply low lights or for fashion colouring.

Preparation of tints for application

Once the incompatibility test, strand test and test cutting have been carried out successfully it is possible to continue with the colouring process. Where, on Caucasian hair, it may be possible to achieve 2 lifts with 30 vol. or 9%, on African-Caribbean hair you may not achieve the true target colour with the same strength of peroxide because of the natural depth of the base shade. It may be necessary to go one strength up. This is only advisable, however, for natural hair and should not be carried out on hair which has been chemically treated. Always remember to follow the manufacturer's instructions accurately.

Tints come in tubes or cans. If using tubes, half a tube is usually sufficient for a regrowth application. A full tube may be necessary for a full head application or if the hair is very thick. Be sure to mix the tint with the correct strength hydrogen peroxide, following the manufacturer's instructions. Blend the two together using a tint brush. Tints should only be mixed prior to application.

Virgin hair application

1 Ensure the client is adequately covered with a tinting gown and appropriate towel.
2 It is advisable not to shampoo hair prior to tinting as the natural oils produced on the scalp will act as a protective barrier against possible sensitisation. However, if the hair is saturated with heavy oils one shampoo can be administered, taking care to avoid over-stimulating the scalp.
3 Divide the hair into four sections (see page 41).

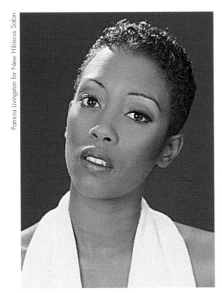

Permanent hair colour

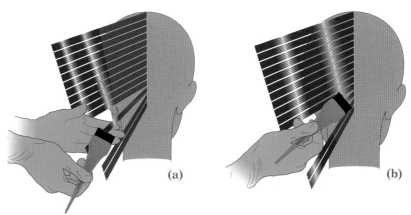

(a) Tint being applied from mid lengths to ends; (b) Tint being applied to root area

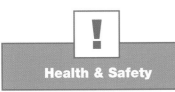

Health & Safety

If another chemical service is evident on the hair or if the client intends to wear a relaxer or permanent wave in the near future, please ensure that the hair is relaxed or permanent waved first and that there is no regrowth showing. If permanent colour is applied to hair which has a regrowth area then breakage may occur when carrying out subsequent relaxing/permanent wave processes as this will overlap the previous colouring service.

Tip

The client should be advised to use an aftercare shampoo specifically designed for colour-treated hair in order to avoid colour fade.

4   Mix the tint for application. At this stage only mix half the desired amount.

5   Taking 6 mm ($\frac{1}{4}$ inch) partings horizontally, work around the head, applying to mid-lengths to ends first (a).

6   Check manufacturer's instructions to see if heat is required and leave to develop for half the processing time.

7   Prepare the other half of your tint mixture.

8   Apply to the root area and leave to develop for the second half of the processing time (b).

9   If darkening hair, the colour can be applied to the full length of hair in one application.

10   Check the result by wiping off some tint with damp cotton wool.

11   Once the desired result has been achieved, take the client to the shampoo basin and damp the hair with a little tepid water. Tint removes tint so massage the tint at the hairline in order to avoid colour settling on the skin.

12   Shampoo the hair twice, using an acid balanced shampoo in order to close the cuticle. Rinse with an antioxidant rinse to prevent the tint from oxidising any further and to seal the colour.

13   The hair is now ready for styling. Remember to fill out a record card.

Regrowth application

1   Gown the client and section the hair as for a virgin head application.

2   Check the client's record card if the tint was carried out at your salon to ensure exact colour as used previously.

3   If the tint was not carried out at your salon, use hair swatches from the manufacturer's colour chart to guide you in making a decision about the previous colour applied to the hair (a).

4   Proceed with the regrowth application in the same manner as a virgin head application except that tint is applied to the roots only, where the client's natural base colour can be seen (b) & (c).

5   Check the manufacturer's instructions for development time.

6   Once the roots are developed, check the colour at the roots and compare with the rest of the hair to see if you need to blend through to the rest of the hair. Use damp cotton wool to wipe a few strands of hair clean at the root area.

7   If necessary, comb through to ends of hair and leave for 10 minutes.

8   If colour fade on the mid-lengths and ends of the hair is obvious then add an equal amount of tepid water to any remaining tint in the bowl and apply to the rest of the hair. The water dilutes the mixture so that there is no colour lift but it acts more as a semi/quasi-permanent. Alternatively, prepare semi/quasi-permanent mixture and apply to mid-lengths and ends (d).

9   Depending on the degree of the colour fade, leave on the hair for 10–15 minutes.

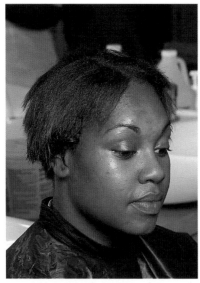

Hair before tint application

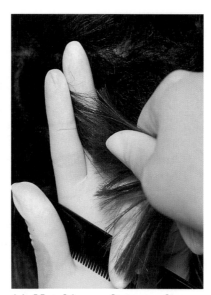

(a) Matching ends to a colour swatch

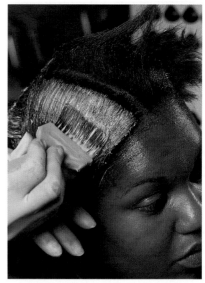

(b) Regrowth colour application

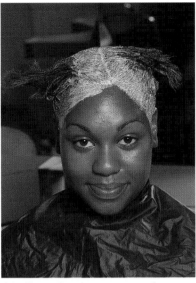

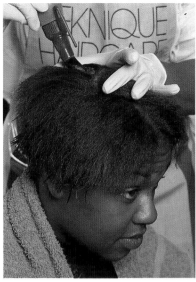

(c) Complete coverage of regrowth area

(d) Quasi colour applied to even out tone

The finished look

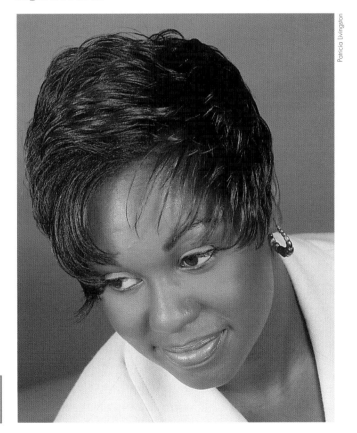

Patricia Livingston

10 If colour fade is excessive, fresh tint should be mixed with equal parts of 6% hydrogen peroxide and applied to the previously colour-treated hair. Leave to process for 10 minutes.

11 Rinse the hair with tepid water and proceed with the shampooing process as for full head application.

12 Fill out a client record card.

Problems encountered during permanent hair colouring

The table outlines problems associated with permanent hair colouring, together with causes and recommended treatment.

Problem	Cause	Treatment
Skin/scalp irritation	Peroxide strength too high; tint still present in hair; hair not shampooed properly; allergic reaction to tint	Shampoo hair thoroughly and advise client to seek medical advice.
Not enough coverage of white hair	Resistant white hair	Apply more product and leave to develop for longer on resistant areas.
Too dark	Incorrect volume of peroxide used (page 187); over-processing when going from light to dark; extremely porous hair	Use colour reducer if necessary (page 214); carry out another tinting application using the correct volume peroxide but only after the hair has been treated.
Too light	Porous hair; peroxide strength too high	Use a darker shade or colour rinse between shampoos.
Too light on ends	Not enough time on comb through	Leave to develop for a further period.
Too much red tone in the hair	Dark natural base	Use a matt or a natural ash colour in the same target colour range to get rid of unwanted red tones.

Bleaching

The term 'bleaching' means the removal of natural pigments (melanin/pheomelanin) from the hair. Bleaching is carried out for two reasons:

1 to lighten hair to a shade which cannot be achieved by using a tint or

2 to pre-lighten hair in preparation for another colour which could be a temporary colour, a semi-permanent colour, a quasi-colour or a permanent colour.

Chemistry

Bleaching is achieved with a mixture of hydrogen peroxide (the oxidising agent) and ammonium hydroxide or

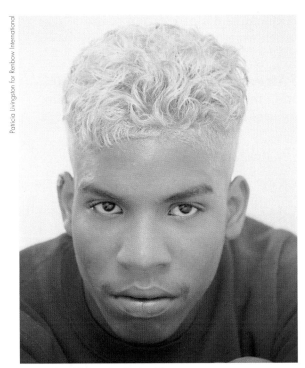

Patricia Livingston for Renbow International

Bleached blonde hair (from a natural base of a 2)

Tip

Bleaching African-Caribbean hair to a white stage is virtually impossible and stressful to the hair. It is important to note that because of the predominant red pigment found in African-Caribbean hair, when the hair is bleached it may appear 'brassy yellow' or 'orange yellow'. If the hair is already chemically processed, it is not wise to carry out more than one application of bleach. However, if it is virgin hair, the effect of white hair can be achieved by bleaching the hair to a level 6 and thereafter using a high lift tint with an ash or violet base.

ammonium carbonate (an alkaline substance). Bleaching African-Caribbean hair is a very delicate process, especially when working with hair which is already chemically processed. It is advisable to use bleach mainly for highlighting purposes or only on short hair when carrying out a full head application.

Bleach, when mixed, is alkaline in composition. The alkaline bleach enters the cortex of the hair, changing the natural darker pigments (eumelanin) to colourless compounds. This takes place by the addition of oxygen to the pigment from the hydrogen peroxide, bringing about an oxidation process.

In African-Caribbean hair, due to the fact that the eumelanin granules are large and widely spaced, it is easier for the bleach to have an effect. However, the lighter pigments (pheomelanin) are small in molecular structure and therefore more resistant to bleach. These pigments are also found in African-Caribbean hair but in smaller quantities than Caucasian hair.

The chemical reaction of bleach and hydrogen peroxide can be shown thus:

melanin	+ oxygen	=	oxymelanin
(black/brown)	(from hydrogen peroxide)		(colourless)
pheomelanin	+ oxygen	=	oxypheomelanin
(red/yellow)	(from hydrogen peroxide)		(colourless)

As mentioned above, black and brown pigments are more easily oxidised and oxidation therefore takes place in three stages:

black/brown → red/yellow → yellow

African-Caribbean hair, when bleached will lighten in this order:

black → brown → red → red-gold → gold → yellow →

pale yellow → (white)

If bleaching is necessary, it is more advisable to carry it out on virgin African-Caribbean hair. If the hair is already chemically treated, then it is likely to be more porous than virgin hair. The effect of bleach on this type of hair will cause the hair to become even more porous, thereby causing damage to the internal structure of the hair. Some bleaching processes may require the hair to have more than one application of bleach to lift the hair up to the

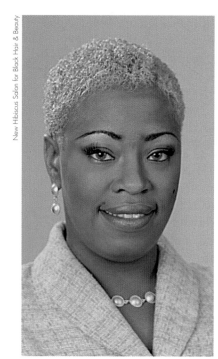

Bleached blonde and toned with gold

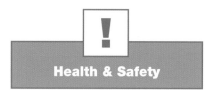

Health & Safety

A strand test should always be carried out beforehand to ascertain whether the hair can withstand the bleaching process.

desired colour. This can cause disintegration of the disulphide bonds to such an extent that permanent damage may occur.

During bleaching of African Carribean hair, almost 50% of the disulphide bonds may be degraded. This weakens the hair considerably and it is therefore unwise to carry out any other chemical services such as a relaxer or curly perm on a client with a high percentage of bleached hair.

Full head application

1   Gown and protect the client with a suitable towel.

2   Protect yourself with apron and gloves.

3   Do not shampoo the hair before bleaching as natural oils on hair and scalp will protect the scalp from sensitisation, especially if more than one application of bleach is necessary. However, in cases where there is heavy usage of moisturising gels, the client must be advised to shampoo her hair at least 2 days prior to bleaching and not to use any more gels until after the bleaching service.

4   Divide hair into four sections, from ear to ear and forehead to nape.

5   Apply barrier cream to the hairline and over the ears.

6   Mix the bleach following the manufacturer's instructions. The bleach should not be allowed to stand but should be used immediately following mixing.

7   Apply bleach to the nape area first which tends to be the most resistant part of the head.

8   A full head of bleach application to virgin hair is carried out in the same manner as that for tinting, i.e. apply mid-lengths to ends then roots (page 199).

9   Always use an adequate amount of bleach and take smaller sections than when tinting because the smallest area left uncovered will show up.

10   Cross check application thoroughly.

11   Leave to develop until half way through the desired time then apply to the root area and leave to develop for the second half of the time. The body heat from the client should speed up the bleaching process on the root area.

12   Once the correct colour has been achieved, rinse with tepid water and shampoo with an acidic shampoo.

13   Follow through with an antioxidant rinse to neutralise the alkalinity of the bleach and to prevent further

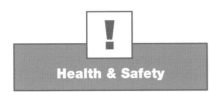

Remember to conduct all necessary tests before deciding to carry out any bleaching techniques to the hair. If the hair is over 50 mm (2 inches) long and already chemically processed with a relaxer or permanent wave, then it is not advisable to carry out a full head bleaching application.

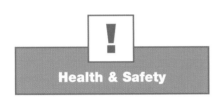

If any bleach has come into contact with the client's skin, remove it immediately. If any bleach gets into the client's eyes, flush immediately with running water.

oxidation. This would prevent any traces of bleach left in the cortex from causing creeping oxidation – the antioxidant rinse gives off hydrogen which will connect with any oxygen from the bleach to form water (H_2O).

14   The hair is now ready for toning if necessary. Toning will get rid of any unwanted hair colour. Remember, yellow is one of the hardest pigments to get rid off so if there are unwanted yellow tones in the bleached hair, they can be neutralised with violet.

Regrowth application

1   Follow safety procedures as with a full head application.
2   Apply bleach to regrowth only.
3   Make sure that the colour on the root matches the colour on the rest of the hair.
4   Remove bleach as for full head application and apply toner if necessary. Style as desired.

Development time

Consult the manufacturer's instructions about timing the bleaching process. However, do bear in mind that extreme salon temperature conditions can affect the timing, as can hair which is porous. Do not leave your client during the bleaching process and constantly check development by removing bleach from a few strands of hair using cotton wool and warm water. Some bleaches are blue in colour and may give an incorrect reading in certain lighting conditions.

Fashion techniques

Once you have mastered the art of bleaching, there are many exciting ways to enhance a hairstyle with the addition of bleach. Always envisage the finished hairstyle then decide where bleaching would be most effective.

Scrunching

This type of colouring is more effective on a curly perm where the hair has been cut into a short style. The ends are dappled with bleach to add more interest to the style. The consistency of the bleach must be thick so that it does not run.

Tip

Care must be taken when working with bleach products as they have a tendency to expand during processing and can cause seepage.

1 Wearing gloves, apply bleach with the fingertips to the ends of the hair.

2 Once the processing time is over, shampoo the hair and proceed with styling or applying other colour products if necessary.

Highlighting and lowlighting

Highlighting using bleach or tint and lowlighting are both effective ways of colouring African-Caribbean hair. They allow you to control the amount of hair which will be colour-treated and can be a good introduction to a client considering full head colour. Highlighting and lowlighting can be carried out by using one of two methods, cap or foil/meche.

The term lowlights was used originally to describe the addition of tone or the darkening of the hair using tint. Nowadays 'lowlighting' refers to both the addition of tone and the lightening of hair using tint.

Hair can also be highlighted using bleach or hilift tint. Bleach will produce rapid lift, allowing the hair to be lightened to a platinum blonde shade, if necessary, depending on the hair type. As mentioned before, bleach can damage the hair and must be used carefully and only on hair in a very good condition. Alternatively hilift tint can be used on hair of a base 5 and lighter for the best results. Hilift tint can produce a variety of blonde shades with differing tones. It should be noted that this type of product is less damaging on the hair than bleach and is possibly better suited to chemically processed hair, particularly when trying to achieve blonde shades.

Lightening the hair using tint will lift the hair up to three shades lighter and add tones such as copper, burgundy and mahogany. Ultimately the use of tint on African-Caribbean hair to lighten and add tone is kinder and less damaging, than hilift tint or bleach.

Cap method

When cap highlighting or lowlighting, always ensure that the holes in the cap have not become too large with previous use, otherwise seepage may take place. If the hair is coated with gel or heavy oils, it would be advisable to use a gentle cleansing shampoo to cleanse the hair before beginning the process, but otherwise it is not necessary to shampoo the hair.

Tip

To make fitting of the highlighting cap easier, sprinkle a little talcum powder inside the cap.

Tip

Pulling through more strands of hair will result in stronger highlights. Fewer strands will give a more subtle effect.

Procedure

1 Gown and protect the client with a towel.

2 Shampoo the hair if necessary and dry it entirely before starting.

3 Comb all the hair back to allow the cap to be fitted with ease.

4 Check the hairline first to ensure that there is no previous history of breakage. If there is, do not pull any strands of hair through from the hairline.

5 Using a crochet hook, start at the outer edge of the cap and pull strands of hair through holes in the cap until you have pulled through sufficient hair for highlighting (a).

6 Once you are satisfied that enough hair has been pulled through, mix the bleach or tint. Do not mix beforehand otherwise the mixture will oxidise and therefore lose some of its strength.

7 Apply the tint (b).

8 Monitor the development of the colour and remove as soon as the desired colour is achieved (c).

9 Rinse the hair thoroughly until all excess colour is removed (d).

10 Apply conditioner to colour treated hair before removing the cap. This will make removing the cap eaier and avoid pulling on the hair or scalp (e).

11 Remove the cap holding the roots of the hair to avoid pulling the scalp (f).

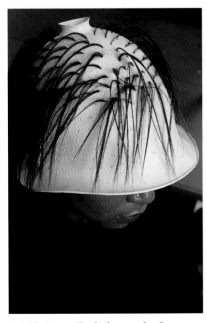

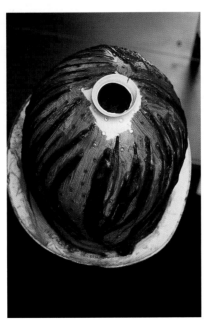

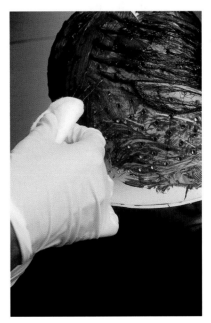

(a) Hair pulled through the cap   (b) Applying tint   (c) Checking colour result

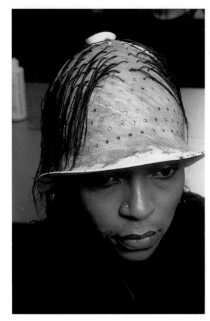

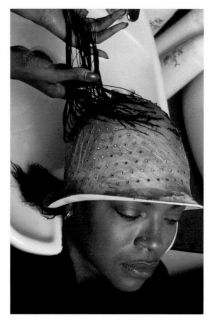

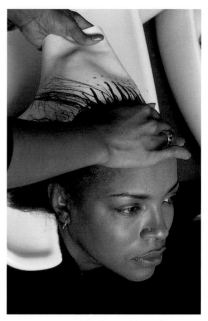

(d) Colour after rinsing

(e) Conditioner applied to make cap removal easier

(f) Removing the cap holding the roots of the hair to avoid pulling the scalp

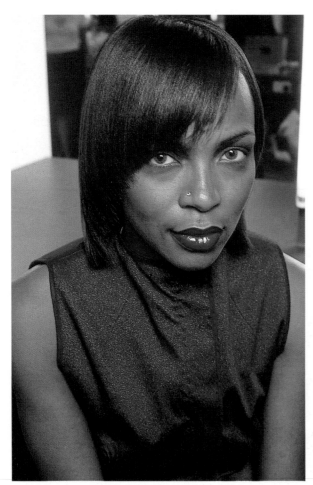

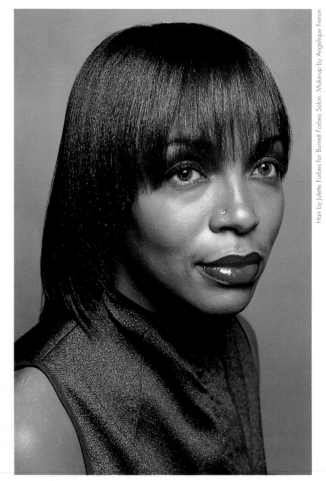

The finished style

Hair by Juliette Forbes for Burnett Forbes Salon. Make-up by Angelique Ferron

Foil method

This method of highlighting or lowlighting is time-consuming but there are added benefits in that you are able to work closer to the scalp than with the cap method. Also, you are able to see exactly where the highlights are being placed on the head. Foil or self-adhesive strips (meche) are used to keep hair for highlighting in place. Hair is separated using a pintail comb with a weaving technique.

A systematic approach is necessary when working with foil/meche highlights. It is best to use the nine section method as described on page 124.

Procedure

1   Cut strips of foil about 100 mm (4 inches) wide and to the length of the hair you will be working with.

2   Place the foil shiny side down and fold along the top edge to create a lip 6 mm ($\frac{1}{4}$ inch) wide. This allows you to place the pintail end of the comb inside the lip of foil and gives a more secure edge to work with.

3   Prepare the bleach/colourant according to the manufacturer's instructions. Do not mix too much product at this stage because it is a lengthy process and the product may oxidise.

4   Weave the hair with the pintail comb and place a weaved section on the foil. Place the folded edge of the foil as close as possible to the scalp with the dull side facing up.

5   Apply the colour mixture with a tinting brush to approximately 6 mm of the folded edge. Do not apply too much product as it will expand during processing and may cause seepage.

6   Seal the foil by folding in half diagonally so that the top and bottom edges meet. Fold the side edges in towards the middle. Then, using the pointed end of the tail comb, press the top edge of the foil packet across the root section to seal it and prevent the packet from slipping off.

7   Continue working up the head until the application is completed. As this is a long process, some of the packets closer to the nape area may have developed before you have finished your application.

8   Constantly check development. Once some of the packets have developed sufficiently, take the client to the shampoo basin, remove the packets and rinse the bleach from the hair, making sure to secure out of the way any packets which are still developing.

Alternatively, open the packets, spray each section with water and remove the bleach with cotton wool. Apply conditioner (anti-oxidant) to ensure the action of any bleach residue is stopped. If tint is being used there is no need to remove the product, as tint will stop processing once it reaches its developing time.

9   Remember not to mix too much bleach at once – you may need to remix, apply and remove when processed.

10   Once the last packets of hair have developed, remove the remaining foil packets and shampoo the hair.

11   Toner can be added at this stage if required (see below).

Tipping

This is similar to highlighting and can be done using either a highlighting cap or foil. In both cases use thicker sections of hair than for highlighting. Tipping is sometimes preferred to highlighting as it is only the ends of the hair which are treated with the bleach mixture.

Procedure

1   Gown and protect the client with a towel.

2   Put on protective gloves.

3   Mix the colourant and apply to the tips with the fingers. If the hair is long, wrap individual sections in foil to avoid seepage.

4   Check development and remove when processed.

Toning

If the client requires a bleach toner, choose a suitable colour with her. Remember, on darker skins a pale yellow depth will look too brassy so apply an ash toner for a more matt effect.

1   If applying toner to cap highlights, do not remove the cap.

2   Apply the toner but remember that the hair is very porous at this stage so use either a 10 vol./3% peroxide to mix with the toner as the hair will grab the toning product quickly.

3   Continually monitor the development of a bleach toner. Once it is ready, rinse off immediately as it will be difficult to remove colour which has grabbed too much (see page 214).

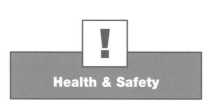

Health & Safety

It is advisable to carry out a tensile strength test whilst checking the degree of lightness as this will indicate the amount of elasticity in the hair and whether the process should be continued (see Chapter 2).

4   Lay the section you are checking over a fresh piece of cotton wool and check the degree of lightness obtained. If the hair is not light enough, reapply bleach and leave to develop.

Block colouring

When block colouring, it is best to look at the finished style and decide where colour should be applied to maximise the effect:

- On layered hair, a section around the front hairline can be coloured so that when the hair is styled off the face the colour can be seen but when it is styled on the face, the colour will diffuse through the rest of the hair which falls on top.
- More interest can be added to a graduated cut by colouring the shorter hair in the nape a different colour to the longer lengths of hair.
- On long hair, block colouring can take place on a lock of hair which can be styled off the face, with a side or centre parting. If the client normally wears her hair in a centre parting, ensure that equal sections of colour fall either side of the parting.

General hints related to bleaching

Removal of bleach products

1   Remove any bleach product by rinsing with warm water until it runs clear.
2   Give one or two shampoos according to the manufacturer's instructions, taking care not to irritate the scalp, especially if more than one application of bleach has been given.
3   Apply antioxidant conditioner, rinse and style as desired.

Additional heat source

It is possible to use an additional heat source when bleaching, such as a steamer or accelerator. This cuts the development time in half.

Conditioning

An antioxidant acid rinse may be used to ensure all activity of the bleach has been stopped. However, do bear in mind that the hair will be more porous at this stage so extra conditioning may be necessary.

Gently squeeze water from hair and apply conditioner or a restructurant.

Problems encountered during bleaching

The table below outlines some problems related to bleaching, together with possible causes.

Problem	Cause
Skin/scalp irritation	• not using barrier cream around the hairline • volume of hydrogen peroxide too high for client's skin • bleach left on too long
Hair breakage/damage	• failure to carry out a strand test (see page 186) • overlapping bleach onto previously bleached hair • bleach applied to hair which has recently undergone another chemical process (relaxer or perm) • volume of hydrogen peroxide too high (see page 187) • bleach left on too long
Hair not light enough	• incorrect analysis of natural hair colour, depth and tone • bleach oxidised by mixing too soon and losing its strength • development time not long enough.
Hair too light	• incorrect analysis of natural hair colour, depth and tone • development time too long
Uneven colour	• not enough product used • uneven application of bleach • application not cross checked properly • incorrect application of large regrowth

Colour correction

Colour correction is usually carried out if the client is unhappy with the end result of the colouring process. This could occur as a result of:

● hair coming out too light

● hair not light enough – check tensile strength before attempting to gain a lighter colour

● unwanted tones.

Before attempting to carry out any form of colour correction, make sure that the hair can withstand another colouring service. Often clients will insist that this be done on the same day. Tell the client what the options are but in no way risk carrying out another service which will jeopardise the condition of the hair. Consult with the client again as to the target colour to be achieved.

Colour restoration

Colour restoration is carried out if the colour has faded or if the hair is too light for the client. In the case of the latter, the client may want to return to her original colour or several shades darker. This can be achieved by a process called pre-pigmentation.

Pre-pigmentation

Bleaching removes the natural pigments from the hair. In order to reverse this action, the colour molecules which have been removed have to be replaced, otherwise the colour may look flat or, even worse, appear to have a greenish tinge. Lost pigment can be restored using either semi-permanent colourants, quasi-permanent colourants or tints. If tint is applied, do not mix with hydrogen peroxide but with a little water, usually two parts water to one part tint.

Final target colour = 1–3; filler colour = red mix.

Final target colour = 4–5; filler colour = 5 R (red).

Final target colour = 6–7; filler colour = 7 (Copper/Copper Gold).

Final target colour = 8–10; filler colour = G mix.

(Target numbers refer to the ICC shade chart.)

Application

1 Apply pre-pigmentation to bleached/faded areas evenly using a tint brush. Keep colour well away from any hair which is not to be pre-pigmented.
2 Blot pre-pigmented area and apply target colour using 20 vol./6% peroxide.
3 Leave for 20–30 minutes.
4 Remove and style as desired.

Reduction of colourants

This process is carried out if a client wants a tint removed or lightened. Colour reducing can be achieved by using either:

- a bleach-based product or
- a ready made product.

Bleach-based products will tend to strip out unwanted colour along with some of the hair's natural pigment. This is not suitable for African-Caribbean hair which is already chemically treated with either a relaxer or a perm, especially where full head application of colour reduction product is necessary.

Ready made colour reducers are made of sodium bisulphite or sodium formaldehyde sulphoxylate. They break down the artificial colours locked into the hair during the tinting process into smaller molecules so that they are easily washed out. These products should not be used to remove colour from chemically relaxed or permed hair.

Colour reducing products will not reverse the bleaching effects of pre-lightening the hair, nor will they restore hair to its original colour. They will, however, prepare the hair to accept another colour if the first colour is unsuitable. When all the artificial colour has been rinsed away, a new tint can be applied to the desired target colour. In all cases check manufacturer's instructions for application procedure and removal.

Hair extensions

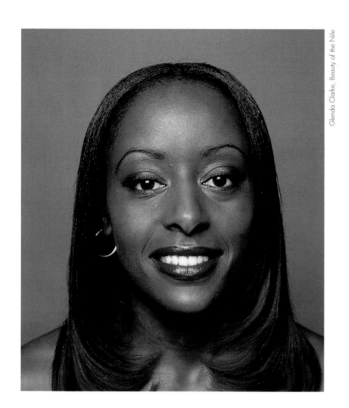

12

Glenda Clarke, Beauty of the Nile

Learning objectives

This chapter covers the following:

- Consultation and analysis
- Cane row extensions
- Single plaits extensions
- Fashion locks
- Weaving
- Sewn/stitched weave
- Natural weave parting

- Bonding
- Partial head weave
- Laser weave
- Micro bonding
- Mesh technique
- Cap technique
- Cutting and styling

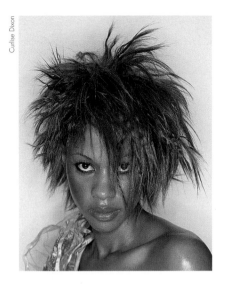

Curtise Dixon

Adding extensions to hair is not a new art form but has been practised for centuries throughout the African diaspora. Both men and women wore extensions in a variety of materials, with some styles taking days to complete due to their elaborate design. Currently, in the more developed parts of Africa, this art form has lost some of its intricate nature. However, in areas such as Papua New Guinea and those unexplored parts of the interiors of Africa, the tradition still continues.

Currently, hair extensions have become so commercialised that they are being used across all cultures – whether it's the more outrageous coloured extensions for fun, subtle pieces to give the appearance of thickness or length or simply to have a complete new look. Hair extensions are carried out on all types of hair whether it is natural or chemically processed. Such is the demand now for hair extensions, that there are salons which cater only for clients requiring extension work.

Consultation and analysis

Consultation must take place before any kind of extension work is carried out. Follow the general procedure for consultation and analysis as described in Chapter 1. In addition, several factors need to be taken into consideration: the client's hair texture, hair length, whether the hair is natural/virgin or chemically processed, the client's face shape, the desired style to be achieved (whether it is plaiting or weaving), the type of extension to be used and any contraindications relating to the client's scalp/hair. These are also discussed in more detail in Chapters 1, 2, 6 and 15.

Hair texture

African-Caribbean hair has three main different textures: fine, medium and coarse, with variations in between such as fine to medium texture and medium to coarse texture (see Chapter 2 for more information).

When working on fine hair, precaution should be taken so that any extension work does not put too much strain on the client's natural hair thereby causing stress points. In addition, hair texture needs to be taken into consideration because during extension work such as weaving, the weave needs to look as natural as possible and the type of extension chosen should be close to the client's own hair texture. This is not to say that other textures cannot be used. Some styles are better achieved using a particular type of extension hair – for example, if the style has a lot of volume, it would be better to use a more coarse textured hair otherwise the hair would lie too flat.

Hair length

Hair length is important for several reasons:-

1   If the client's hair is very short, plaiting may be difficult and, even if it is possible to plait the hair, the life span of it may be limited. When working on long hair, and if plaiting is being carried out, it is necessary to ensure that the extension hair goes beyond the client's own hair to make allowances for securing the ends of the hair whether by burning the ends, attaching beads, knotting the ends or leaving the ends to fall free when using curly extensions or human hair.

2   When stitch weaving, if the client's own hair is short and a sewn weave is required, it would be best to use extension hair to put in a cane rowed base, thereby securing the short hair within the extension hair. If this is not done, and the client's hair is cane rowed without extension, there is a possibility that the canerow will unravel over a period of time, thereby affecting the longevity of the weave. Otherwise, it may be better to suggest the bonding technique as described later in this chapter.

3   Long hair poses a different problem. If the client desires a stitched weave, it is important that the client's own hair is cane rowed fairly small with or without extensions, otherwise it would look too bulky and the weave would not sit flat on the head. Again, it is important that on long hair, the ends of the hair are positioned in such a way that they do not create too much bulk when the extension hair is stitched to it.

Natural/virgin or chemically processed hair

If the client's hair is natural, it is advisable to blow dry the hair first before attaching the extensions. Blow drying will stretch the natural hair, making it easier to work with. With natural/virgin hair, the client's options for extensions are somewhat limited.

For cane rowing and plaiting, once the client's hair is blow-dried, any type of extension hair can be used. However, for durability and longevity of style, it is advisable to use a slightly coarse grade of synthetic hair. Any other type of extension could look untidy after a few weeks if the natural hair, which has been blow-dried prior to extensions, starts to revert. This will be particularly unsightly if human hair has been used for the extension work.

For weaving, again any type of weft hair can be used as long as none of the client's hair is to be left out. If it is, then the client has to be made aware that the hair which has been left out will revert. To avoid this, the client can opt for regularly thermal styling of the hair which is exposed, or chemically relaxing these areas (if necessary) to blend in with the texture of the extension hair. This often defeats the object of having natural hair as part will be chemically processed. When the extensions have been removed this poses a problem because most of the hair is natural and part of it chemically processed.

Bonding on natural hair can be carried out as a temporary style. However, because bonding allows the client's hair to be exposed as bonded strips are attached to the base of the hair close to the scalp, it is important that the client's hair is blow-dried and thermal pressed prior to extension work. If not, the natural hair will be too bulky for extension hair, unless a similar textured hair is being used for the extension work which will enable the client's hair and the extension hair to blend in together.

Chemically processed hair can be cane rowed, plaited, woven or bonded without problems. The only consideration to be given is if the client's hair is relaxed and a curly weave is being attached whilst leaving some of the client's hair out (for example, around the hairline). This can be overcome by using a moisturising gel, brushing the relaxed areas flat and styling the curly weave as desired. If, however, the client's own hair is long and hair is left out around the hairline, it may be difficult to conceal the relaxed hair by gelling it and brushing. This will have to be discussed with the client and an alternative style sought.

A similar problem is encountered when working with relaxed hair and using curly bulk hair for plaiting. Generally speaking, if curly hair is used for plaiting, it is expected that the hair will only be partially plaited, allowing the natural curl of the extensions to fall free. If the client's hair is short this may not pose too much of a problem, however if it is long, the ends of the client's hair which is relaxed will lie straight in between the curl and will be noticeable because the two textures are different. Again, this will have to be explained to the client before starting.

If the client's hair is curly permed, extensions can be carried out. However, with the exception of bonding, the client has to be advised that it is likely that the curl structure of the perm may loosen once the hair has been blow-dried and cane rowed, plaited or woven. In addition, the maintenance product used whilst wearing any type of extensions apart from bonding tends to be a moisturising agent. If this is not used, the hair and scalp will become very dry and, in the case of curly perms, the hair will become excessively dry. Once any moisturing product is used, however, the permed hair which had been blow-dried will begin to revert and look untidy.

Where bonding is concerned, it is not advisable to carry out this process because the client will need to continue using moisturising products to maintain the curl pattern and this will loosen the bonding.

Face shape

Face shape is important because the client needs the weave to look as natural as possible. Face shape can be oval, round, square, oblong, heart-shaped or diamond and not all styles suit all face shapes. For further information see Chapter 6.

The desired style to be achieved

Most clients opting for extensions have already decided whether they would like their hair cane rowed, single plaited or weaved. There are so many styles available with extensions that it is not possible to detail them all. The options are numerous: clients with short hair can opt for short, medium or long extensions and clients with long hair can opt for short, medium or even longer hair extensions.

It is advisable to note that clients with long hair who would like a change to short hair can only opt for a stitched weave, where all their hair has been cane rowed and the weave attached. If any hair is to be left out at all, whether they are having cane rows, braids, a stitched weave or bonding, the extension hair has to go beyond their own hair so as to avoid cutting the client's own hair during the finishing process.

Type of extension

In the Western world, hair extensions have only become popular in about the last 35 years. Initially only a type of yak hair was used for the extension work but more recently

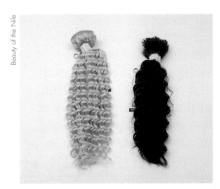

Curly human hair for plaiting or weaving

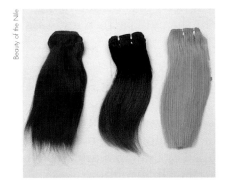

Coloured weft hair for weaving

there has been an explosion of materials, hair types, colours and lengths for extensions, meaning that styles have once more become varied and elaborate. Materials now used for extensions can either be wool/yarn which is used for styles such as fashion locks, human hair or synthetic hair which is made out of nylon. With both synthetic and human hair there is variety in texture such as straight, wavy or curly and they can either be bulk hair for plaiting/cane rowing or weft hair for weaving/bonding.

Contraindications

Contraindications are anything relating to the hair or scalp which would prevent hair extensions from being carried out. This could range from severe hair breakage/hair loss, thinning hair/bald patches which would require particular methods of weaving, or scalp disorders. In some cases where damage is severe, or the scalp is infectious, hair extensions should not be carried out and the client should be advised to seek medical advice.

Hair preparation prior to extension work

Prior to all extension work the hair should be shampooed, conditioned (preferably a deep penetrating, moisturising treatment) and then blow-dried. A light moisturising oil/hairdressing can be applied to the scalp at this stage or at the end of putting in the extensions. When carrying out bonding extensions do not apply any oil to the hair or scalp before or after blow-drying as this will make the base too slippery to work with and the bonding glue will not be as effective. (See Chapters 3 and 5 for more information on shampooing/conditioning and blow-drying.)

Cane row

Cane row, sometimes called corn row, originated in Africa where the technique has been used to create a number of intricate styles. Cane rowing is designed by working along channels of hair and is carried out using three subsections of hair. It can be woven under or over. There are different techniques for starting off the cane row, however the simplest and most effective way is to divide the extension hair into three sections, and place them section for section with the client's own natural hair, which also should be subdivided into three sections at the start of the cane row. The technique carried out below uses synthetic hair.

Technique

1 Shampoo, condition and blow dry hair.

2 Section the client's hair bearing in mind the desired style to be achieved (a). Use section clips to hold the rest of the hair out of the way.

3 Take two sections of extension hair, according to how thick or thin the cane rows are to be. Loop one section over the middle of the other section so that there are three sections (b).

4 Subdivide the client's hair into three sections and line up extension hair, section for section, with client's own hair.

5 Hold the right sections of hair in the right hand between the middle and third fingers whilst holding the middle strands in the right hand between the index finger and third finger. Then hold the left strands between the third and fourth fingers, looping the ends over the thumbs.

6 Place the left index finger under the right index finger and middle strands (c).

7 Pick up the right strands along with some of the client's hair with the left index finger drawing it across under the middle strand into the left hand and holding it between the left index finger and third finger. The middle strands are now transferred to the right hand between the third and fourth fingers, leaving the right index finger to cross under the left index finger and what has now become the middle strands (d).

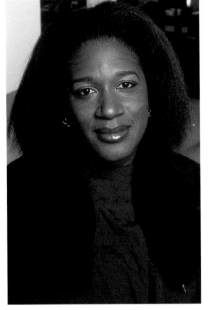

Before

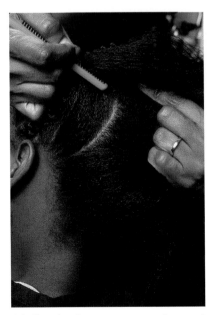

(a) Sectioning cane row channel

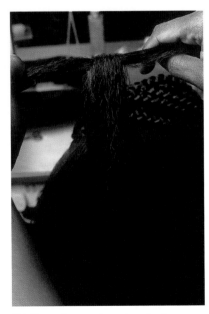

(b) Looping extension hair

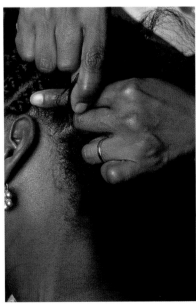

(c) Subdividing the hair and adding extension hair

Health & Safety

Whilst cane rowing, care must be taken not to use too much tension, especially around the hairline, as this could cause traction alopecia.

Tip

For equipment needed, aftercare, shampooing/ conditioning and removal for all techniques see the equipment and maintenance table at the end of this chapter.

The finished style

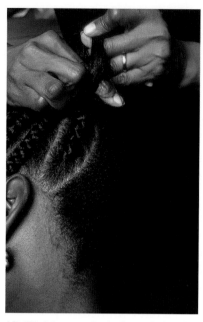 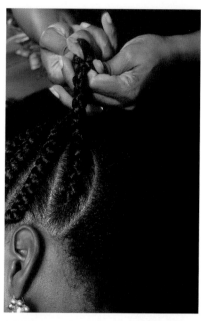

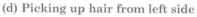

(d) Picking up hair from left side   (e) Three stemmed plait finish

8 Continue crossing under, working along a channel of cane row, pick up more of the client's hair along the channel as each section is taken up. Continue this until the end of the cane row is reached.

9 Finish the cane rowed channel with a three stemmed plait (e).

10 When all is completed, the plaits can be styled as desired.

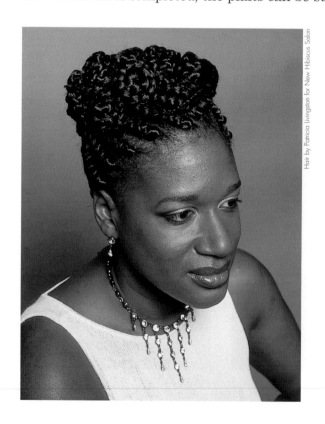

Hair by Patricia Livingston for New Hibiscus Salon

If cane row is being done in an over plaiting technique instead of under, the same applies except that the hair is taken over rather than under.

Single plaits

Like cane rowing, plaiting was a styling technique practised by Africans and it was worn by both men and women.

Plaiting can be carried out on natural or chemically processed hair using synthetic or human extensions, and these can either be straight, wavy or curly. Single plaits are generally added to give the client a new look, longer hair, to allow the hair to have a rest period from chemicals or to aid the client who wishes to go from chemical processing to natural hair.

Once single plaits are added, it is advisable not to leave them in for too long as this could create matting at the root of the hair. An average time for the duration of single plaits is between 6 and 12 weeks. This is not to say that it could not be taken out sooner, but on average the extension should not begin to look untidy for at least one month. Having said this, one has to bear in mind the type of extension hair which has been used. Synthetic hair, which is more coarse in texture, is the type of extension which would last longest as it is generally burnt at the ends to seal it and therefore does not unravel so easily.

Special care must be taken when plaiting hair which has been treated with a curly perm or body wave product. This hair would have been blow-dried prior to plaiting and once permed hair has been blow-dried and hair extensions attached, the curl pattern can become distorted and loosen significantly. Ideally, one should avoid plaiting this hair type. If it is necessary to do so, the client must be informed that if any liquid product is applied to the hair or if the hair is shampooed, the permed hair will begin to revert and will no longer sit straight inside the extension. This could make the appearance very untidy.

Technique

1 Shampoo, condition and blow-dry hair.
2 Starting at the nape, section hair horizontally and secure the rest of the hair out of the way.
3 Divide this horizontal section into smaller square sections and attach extension hair to each of the square sections of the client's hair using the same technique as

Health & Safety

When working around the hairline, make sure that plaits are not too tight otherwise this could cause traction alopecia. Also, ensure that the sections of hair are not too small otherwise the weight of the extension hair may be too heavy for the section of hair and this can create hair loss around the hairline.

Tip

Remember, for aftercare, shampooing/conditioning and removal of single plaits see the maintenance table at the end of this chapter.

described above for cane row extensions – the only difference being that once the extension hair is attached, the hair is plaited as a three stemmed plait rather than worked along a channel as in the cane rows described above (a) and (b).

4   Continue working up the head horizontally, adding extensions until the whole head is completed. For continuity, ensure that each horizontal section is the same size and that each square section of hair is the same size.

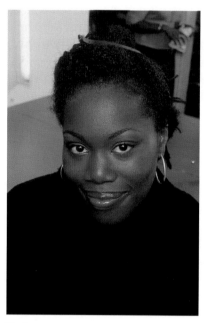

Before

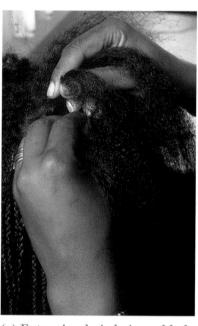

(a) Extension hair being added to client's hair

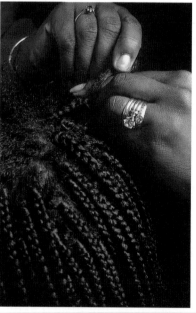

(b)Three stemmed plait

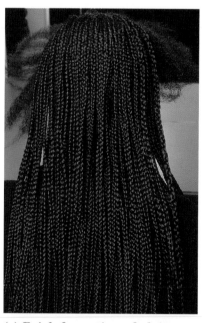

(c) Brick formation of plaits

The finished style

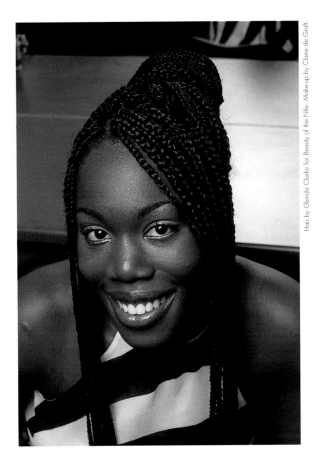

Hair by Glenda Clarke for Beauty of the Nile. Makeup by Claire de Graft.

5   Place each square section of plaits in a brick formation so as not to reveal too much of the scalp and to give the hair a fuller appearance (c).

6   Continue adding extensions until the whole head is completed.

Fashion locks

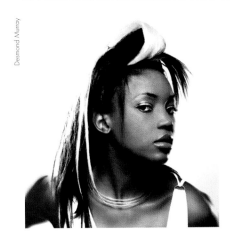

Desmond Murray

Fashion locks are similar to dreadlocks in many ways, which were popularised by the Rastafarian movement back in the 1970s. Dreadlocks involved not shampooing or combing the hair but allowing it to matt and lock as the growing strands of hair intertwine themselves round each other. This concept of locking hair was viewed with some trepidation by the mainstream black populace who did not like the idea of the hair not being shampooed or combed.

However, throughout the 1980s and 1990s the idea of locking hair became more appealing as the process by which locks could be achieved and maintained changed. New techniques and products for locking hair meant that locks could be groomed, unlike their original counterpart where hair was left to grow and fuse together. This new type of lock was not seen by Rastafarians as true locks, but as fashion locks or designer locks.

Fashion locks can be achieved by using a variety of products such as yarn extensions, beeswax, gel, honey or rachet. The locking process starts by twisting the client's natural hair using a single twisting method (see Chapter 13 for the technique) and advising the client to visit the salon periodically to continue the twisting process in the root area as the hair grows. During this period, the hair should not be shampooed until the locking process has taken place. Once this has been achieved, the client must be encouraged to return to the salon at least once a month to separate the locks and retwist the root area.

Alternatively, the hair can be plaited with yarn/wool for a dreadlocks effect. Wool has a dull, dense look to it which resembles that of locks and, once plaited, it can then be wrapped with additional wool to give it a more compact look. This style is suitable for someone who wants a dreadlocks look and does not want to wait the necessary time for their own hair to begin to lock. It can be achieved on natural hair or chemically processed hair. With this style, the client has the best of both worlds – they can have a dreadlocks lookalike straight away whilst still cultivating locks to their own hair.

With the wool technique, the client must be advised to return to the salon after 6–8 weeks so that any new hair which is growing in the root area can be twisted, thus starting off the locking process in their own hair. With each visit to the salon, the hair must be separated at the root and retwisted, encouraging the growth of individual locks rather than a matted look. By the sixth month most, if not all of the wool can be cut from the nape area or all over if the client so desires. At some point there will be a significant amount of the client's own hair in its twisted shape showing in the root area. At this point it will be necessary to advise the client to cut off the wool extensions.

By the time all of the wool has been cut, fusing should be taking place in each twist. This will be apparent because the twists will not unravel or be able to be combed out, because the strands in the twists would have enmeshed themselves around each other causing fusing. The client must be advised to return to the salon regularly for the maintenance and upkeep of the locks.

The technique shown in the photo uses the wool/yarn method. This has been plaited with yarn of a medium size. Some yarn has a wool and nylon mix, and it is best to plait

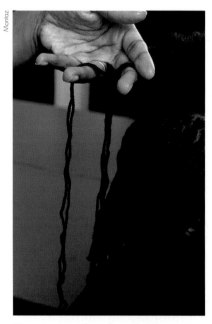

Montaz

Yarn extension for plaiting

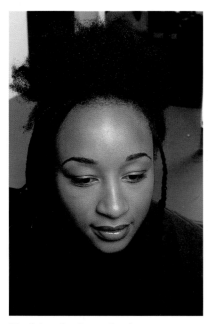

Fashion locks – during application

the hair with this type of yarn because the nylon in the wool allows the ends of the plait to be sealed by burning them.

Technique

1   Shampoo, condition and blow-dry client's hair.
2   Section hair as for single plaiting technique described above (a).
3   Add yarn/wool to client's hair in the form of single plaits following the technique described above (b).
4   As an additional process, one strand of the yarn may be left out during plaiting. This is then used to wrap around the plait and gives a more dense, authentic dreadlocks look.
5   Once extensions are completed, they can be moulded with the fingers.

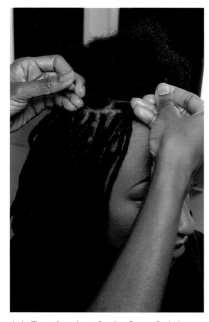

(a) Sectioning hair for plaiting

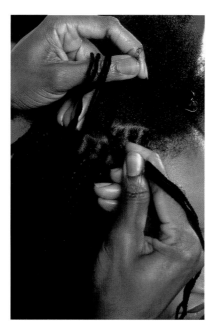

(b) Extension hair being added to client's hair

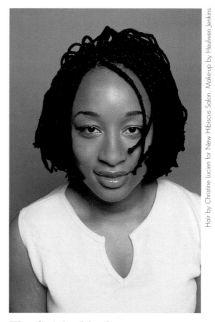

The finished look

Hair by Christine Lucien for New Hibiscus Salon. Make-up by Heulwen Jenkins

Weaving

Weaving first became fashionable in the UK during the 1960s. At that time, yak hair, which produced a bouffant type appearance due to its density, was used for weaving. The yak hair generally did not blend well with most types of African-Caribbean hair and therefore gave a very unnatural look.

Gradually, more sophisticated materials have appeared on the market for weaving. In addition, styling techniques have progressed so much that it is sometimes difficult to identify whether someone is wearing a weave or not.

The idea for weaving originated from the technique used in the production of wigs. Wefts of hair, human or synthetic, are woven into a nylon strip. It is usual to find two strips woven together to create what is known as a weft. The weft has a right and a wrong side and this can easily be detected by looking at it closely where it is stitched to the nylon strip. This weft is then used to sew onto the client's own hair to create a variety of hair styles.

Weaving using a sewing method was the traditional way of doing this and is still quite widely used. It is often preferred to other methods such as bonding (covered later in this chapter) because the extensions are more securely placed as it is sewn to a cane rowed base and it can last longer than other methods, giving better value for money.

If the client's hair is already long and a weave is desired for added thickness, then it is not necessary to carry out a full head weave. Sometimes half a head can be done to create fullness at the back of the head, or sections of the client's own hair can be left free whilst adding extensions to other sections. This is known as a partial weave technique.

When using the sewing technique, the client's hair is generally cane rowed as a base. This base can be cane rowed in different ways and this is dependent mainly on the style to be achieved and the client's own hair length.

Circular base

If the client's natural hair is long, it is better to cane row in a circular fashion so that the end of the cane row can be stitched to the cane rowed hair. To ensure that the weaved extensions last for the optimum time, it is wise to use synthetic extensions to attach to the client's hair whilst forming the cane rowed base. This is especially important if the hair is short, otherwise the cane rowed base may unravel during the life span of the weave, making the weave loose. For the method of attaching synthetic extensions to client's hair to form the cane rowed base see pages 221–2.

Vertical base

Some bases are carried with one circular row around the hairline and the rest of the hair cane rowed vertically. This method is sometimes preferred because once the extension is woven onto the vertical base, it lies flatter than on a circular base. This then tends to make the whole appearance less bulky.

Horizontal base

This is similar in appearance to the circular base except that instead of a continuous circular pattern, the hair is cane rowed horizontally with ends being cane rowed into the next subsection.

Contraindications

If there is noticeable hair loss along the hairline or on the crown, to the extent that the area looks bald, then this would affect the application of the weave, as there will not be any hair to cane row as a base in these areas. This does not mean that someone with this condition cannot have a weave, but an alternative method to a conventional weave has to be used such as the mesh or cap technique, which is described later on in this chapter.

Full head sewn/stitched weave

If the client requires a full head sewn weave with none of their own hair left out, then the whole head must be cane rowed. It is important to point out to the client that styling would be limited: the hair cannot be worn back off the face as this would reveal the mesh of the weave around the hairline. Thus a fringe would need to be worn, or at least there needs to be some hair coming onto the face.

As an alternative, most of the client's own hair can be cane rowed leaving sufficient hair around the hairline free in order to cover the weave if styled upwards or backwards. If this is preferred then the extension hair has to be as close a match as possible to the client's hair, both in colour and texture.

Another option is to stitch weave most of the hair, whilst leaving some of the client's hair free at the crown. Bonded extensions are then added to the rest of the hair. This gives a more natural look. The technique described below is the circular base.

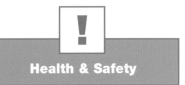

For the less experienced practitioner, a curved needle should be used for weaving to avoid damaging the scalp.

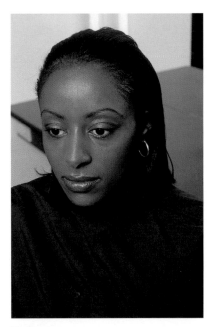

Before

Technique

1   Shampoo, condition and blow dry hair.

2   Starting at the nape, section client's hair for cane rowing (a).

3   Cane row hair using the technique shown earlier in this chapter, bearing in mind the desired finished look. If cane rowing in a circular fashion, ensure that the cane row finishes at the crown of the head. If not, when the weave is sewn on, it will look out of line with the natural contour of the head (b).

4   Thread the needle using only the thread designed for weaving, which is a waxed thread that tends to feel thicker than ordinary thread. If any other thread is used, it will snap easily during sewing or during the life span of the weave. If this happens, the weave extensions will come loose and look unsightly.

5   Measure lengths of weft to hair sections and cut weft (c) and (d).

6   Using the blanket stitching described below, apply weft extension to cane rowed base ensuring that weft is stitched on the right side and not the wrong side.

7   Continue working up the head until entire head is covered (e) and (f).

8   Cut and style weave. (See cutting and styling later on in this chapter.)

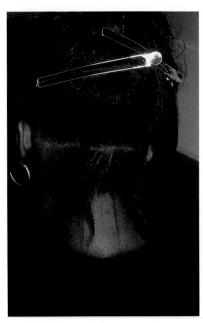

(a) Sectioning at nape

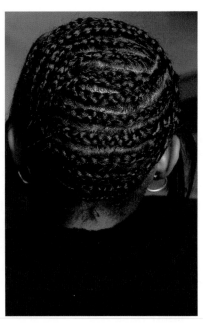

(b) Finished horizontal cane row

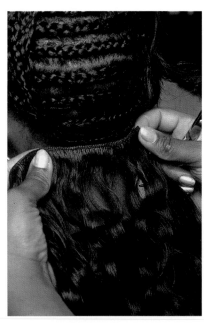

(c) Measuring weft

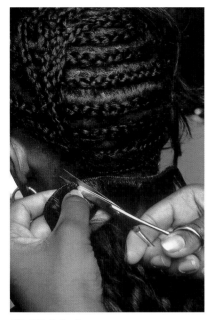

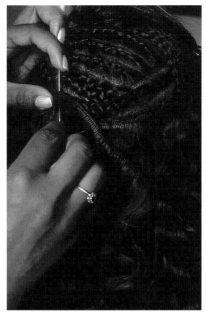

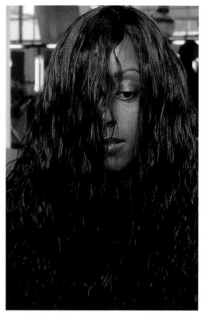

(d) Weft being cut

(e) Attaching wefts to cane row base at the crown

(f) Completed weave

Tip

To blanket stitch, first feed needle through canerowed base and weft, looping needle with each stitch. This ensures that stitching is secure and will not unravel easily.

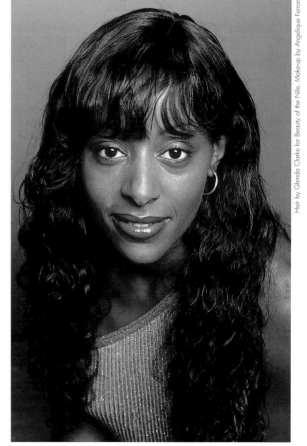

The finished look

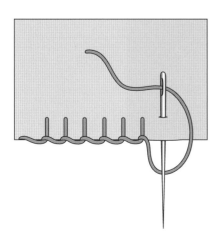

Blanket stitch

Hair by Glenda Clarke for Beauty of the Nile. Make-up by Angelique Ferron.

Natural weave parting

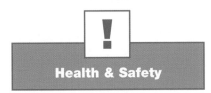
Advise the client not to apply too much force during combing/brushing, as this could put too much stress on the client's own hair and can cause damage.

The natural weave parting was created so as to give the appearance of a parting in the hair, when in reality all of the client's hair has been cane rowed. The natural weave parting is hair attached to a rubber/latex base, which is dyed to give the appearance of the natural tones of the scalp. It is similar to a postiche.

Technique

1   Sew wefts of extension hair to cane rowed base working up to the crown area.

2   Attach natural weave parting to cane rowed base at front of head using sewing technique. It is important that the cane rowed hair underneath is not too bulky, or the natural weave parting will not sit close to the scalp (a).

3   Cut and style weave (b). (See cutting and styling later on in this chapter.)

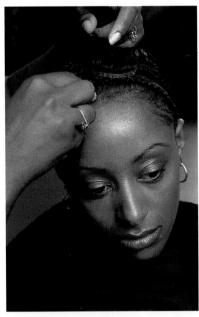

(a) Natural hair parting being sewn in

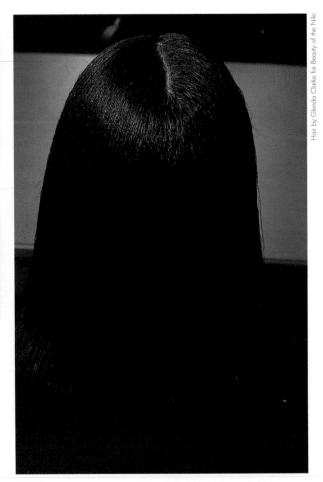

Hair by Glenda Clarke for Beauty of the Nile

(b) Finished style with natural hair parting

Bonding

Bonding is carried out using the same wefts of hair as for sewn weave: it has both advantages and disadvantages. The advantages are that because there is no base to work on, the wefts of extension hair are attached directly to the root of the client's hair and therefore lie flatter on the head than a sewn weave. This gives a more natural appearance to the weave.

The disadvantages are that the bonding technique tends not to last as long as the sewn weave and, if not removed properly, can strip away some of the client's hair during the removal process.

It is more commonplace to carry out bonding on hair which has been chemically processed with a relaxer. If the hair has not been relaxed and is either blow-dried or thermal styled then reversion will take place to the client's own hair and this will eventually be visible through the extension hair as the textures would be different.

Technique

1 Shampoo, condition and blow dry hair – see Chapters 3 and 5. Do not apply any oil-based product at this stage as it will make the surface of the scalp too slippery: wefts will not adhere well to the root area or they will come away quickly.

2 Section hair according to where bonded wefts need to be placed (a).

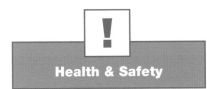

Health & Safety

It is advisable to do a skin test prior to carrying out any bonding work. Apply a small amount of bonding glue to the skin behind the ear and leave for at least 24 hours. If irritation occurs, advise the client to remove the glue with damp cotton wool and inform the salon as soon as possible. Advise the client to seek medical advice if irritation persists.

Tip

Natural/virgin hair, once blow-dried, pressed or tonged, will return to its natural state if it absorbs moisture. This is referred to as reversion.

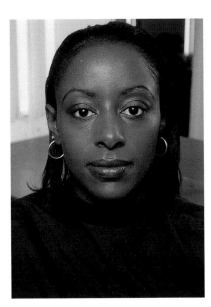

Before

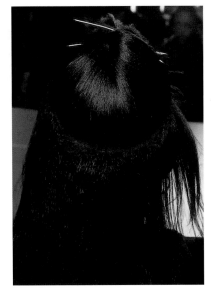

(a) Hair sectioned at nape prior to bonding

3   Measure lengths of weft to hair sections and cut weft. (b)

4   Apply bonding glue to weft strips. For additional hold the glue can also be applied to root of hair close to the scalp (c) and (d).

5   Press weft strips to section of hair where bonding glue has been applied (e).

6   Continue adding weft strips until desired look is achieved.

7   Cut and style. (See cutting and styling later in this chapter.)

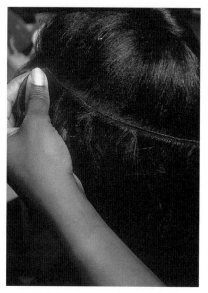

(b) Weft being measured

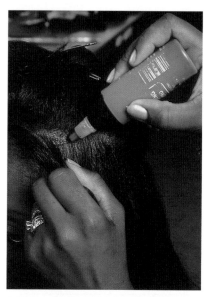

(c) Bonding glue applied to roots of hair

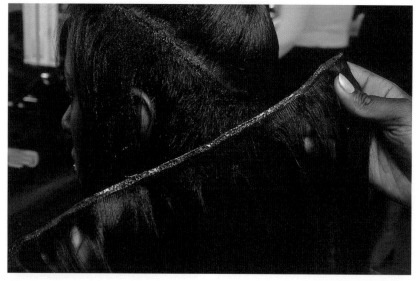

(d) Bonding glue applied to weft

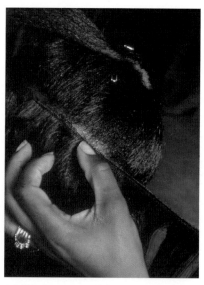

(e) Weft pressed firmly to root area

The finished style

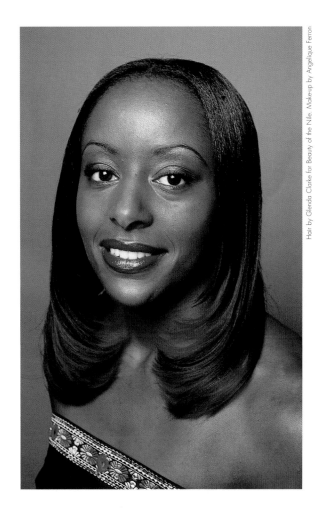

Hair by Glenda Clarke for Beauty of the Nile. Makeup by Angelique Ferron

Partial head weave

This technique is often carried out to add thickness, length or variety to the client's own hair. It is important that the extension hair matches well with the client's own hair, or a contrasting colour can be used to add variety or give the appearance of highlights to the hair. This form of extensions is generally used as a temporary measure and can either be sewn or bonded in. It can be used to extend fringes or hair in the nape area or add fullness or blocks of colour to a hairstyle. The method or technique used depends on the style you want to achieve. The step by step below is one example of this advanced fashion technique used to create a bridal look.

Technique

1   Section the hair where wefts are to be placed and apply first section at front (a).

2 Take a section of client's hair and cover over bonding (b).

3 Section hair at sides and back and apply wefts (c).

4 Cane row crown as a base to create weft ponytail (d).

5 Gather all the hair up into a ponytail and wrap the weft around the hair and cane row, securing it by sewing to the cane rowed base (e).

6 Roller set and style for a bridal look.

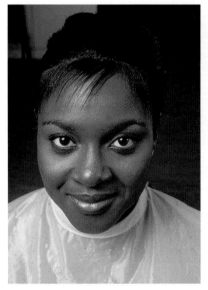

Before

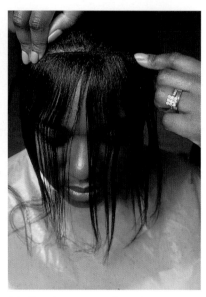

(a) Sectioning and weft application at the front

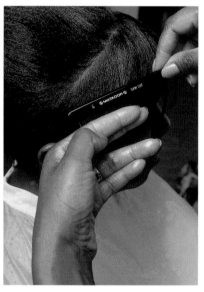

(b) Covering bond extensions with client's hair

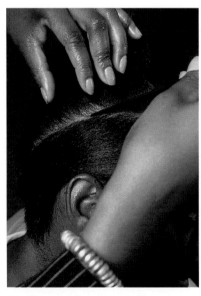

(c) Sectioning for weft application at the sides and back

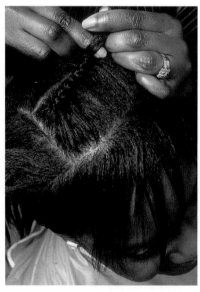

(d) Crown cane rowed as a base for ponytail

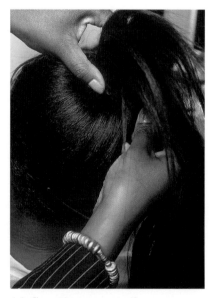

(e) Creating ponytail

A variety of partial weave hairstyles that show the diversity of styles that can be created by using this technique. Each look took between one and a half to two hours to create.

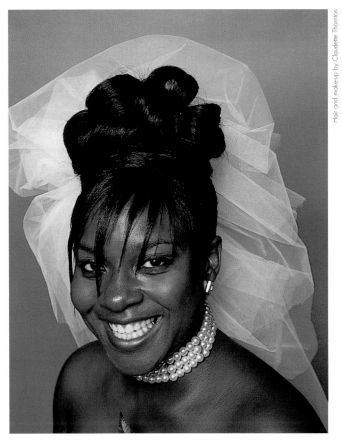

Finished bridal look

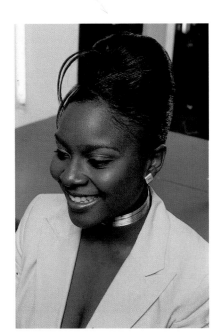

Upswept bouffant look

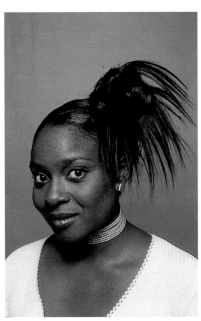

Assymetric spiky look

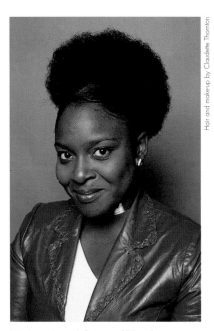

Extension Afro puff look

Laser weave

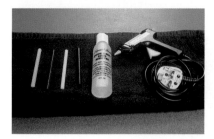

Equipment for laser weave

The laser method of using hair extensions is an application which is considered to be one of the most versatile due to the way it is used. It consists of small quantities of extension hair bonded to small sections of the client's hair; these sections are repeated in a pattern so as to achieve the desired effect. Once applied they can last up to six months, but it is advisable not to leave them on for longer than three months. One of the advantages of wearing a laser weave is that providing due care is taken, it can be shampooed, combed and styled almost in the same way as the client's own hair.

The laser method can only be used on certain textures/types of hair, especially African-Caribbean hair, and should only be carried out by a professional who is fully qualified and trained in this technique. Failure to recognise the different hair types can result in damage/breakage to the hair and even long term damage to the hair follicles.

Technique

1   Shampoo, condition and blow dry the hair into the direction of the style to be achieved. Do not use any oils in the hair or scalp as this can hinder application and cause the hair to slip or adhere insufficiently.

2   Starting just below the occipital bone, section hair horizontally into neat rows, using section clips to keep the rest of the hair out of the way (a).

3   Subdivide the first section into smaller triangular sections (about $\frac{1}{8}$th in area) and without gaps between, thus maximising bulk but minimising bond thickness. Do not apply to the nape area as it is too weak and the

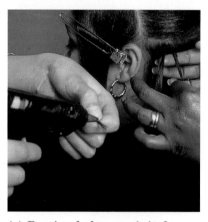

(a) Parting below occipital bone

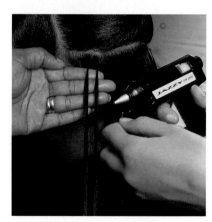

(b) Glue gun for bonding

scalp more tender. In addition, this nape area will cover over any extensions when hair is worn in a ponytail or in an upswept style.

4   Leave sufficient hair all around the hairline – about 2–3 inches – to cover over all extensions. It is important at this stage to ensure that any extension hair to be used is a close match to the existing colour and texture of the client's own hair, otherwise it would look false.

5   Taking extension hair, cut the top to leave the top ends neat. Place glue sticks in electrical glue gun and allow to heat. Apply the hot bonding agent to the extension hair, which is then placed beneath the receiving section of the client's own hair. Care should be taken to avoid overloading the section – the thickness of the extension should never exceed that of the receiving section (b).

6   The extension hair should be applied close to but slightly away from the scalp, thereby avoiding root lift which can cause uneven tension and risk of breakage during brushing (c).

7   Using the fingertips, roll the glue and the extension hair around the receiving section of the client's own hair (d).

8   As each row is completed, check the extensions for mobility in all directions, making sure that any cross hairs which may have inadvertently strayed during the application process are removed. Continue to work up the head in a brick formation so as to minimise gaps.

9   Once all extensions have been completed, carefully brush hair, starting at the ends and working towards the root with an appropriate brush. The hair can then be cut and styled as desired.

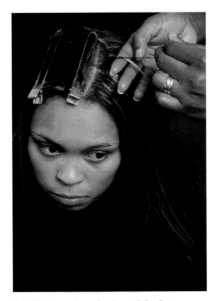

(c) Extension hair added to client's hair

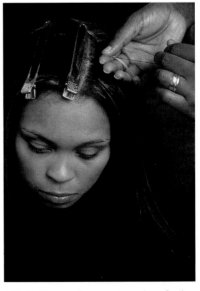

(d) Rolling glue, extension hair and client's hair together

The finished style

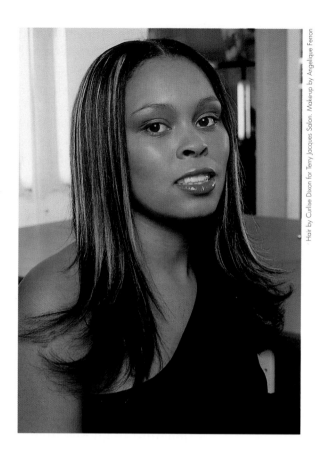

Hair by Curlise Dixon for Terry Jacques Salon. Make-up by Angelique Ferron

The client now has fuller, longer hair which can be shampooed, conditioned, brushed and styled as if it were her own. The client must then be advised to return to the salon every two weeks for maintenance.

Micro bond extensions

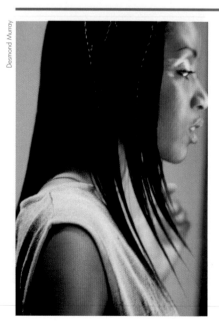

Desmond Murray

An alternative to the laser technique described above is the micro bond. The principles of attaching the extensions are the same (a), (b), (c), (d) & (e). The main difference between this technique and the laser technique is in the removal process. Both techniques use a liquid solvent to soften the seal where extensions have been fused to the client's hair (f). With the micro bond technique, the solvent is made up of a plastic resin which helps to break down the seal to a powdery substance. To assist with the removal, a pair of pinchers is used to crack the seal once the solvent has been placed on the hair (g). This then releases the client's hair from the extension hair.

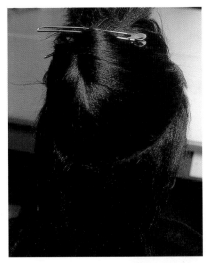

(a) Sectioning at occipital bone

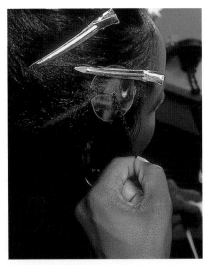

(b) Separate hair prior to bonding

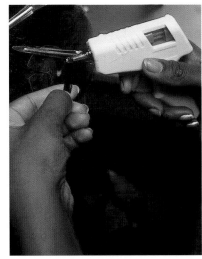

(c) Application of bond solution to extension hair

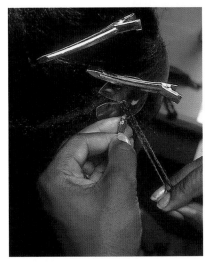

(d) Place extension hair, with bonded tip, against client's hair

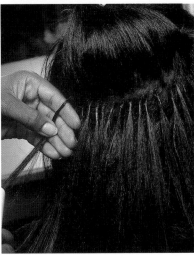

(e) Extensions placed a quarter of an inch apart

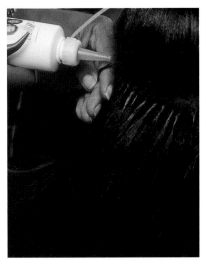

(f) Glue solvent applied to micro strands

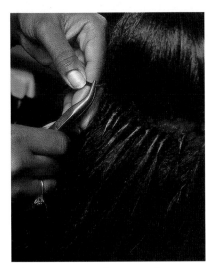

(g) Pincers used to crack microbond seal

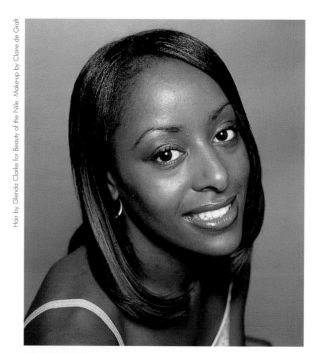

Hair by Glenda Clarke for Beauty of the Nile. Makeup by Claire de Graft

The finished style

Extensions using mesh base

This type of extension is carried out using a hair net. The advantage of this is that if the client's own hair is sparse, the net can act as a base to sew on and therefore cover thinning hair. The disadvantage is that shampooing is more difficult as it will not be easy to massage the scalp because of the net.

The client's hair can either be cane rowed or wrap set before application of the net and the weft extensions can either be stitched or bonded to the net. It is not advisable to keep this type of extension in for a long period of time as the hair and scalp will become very dry and dirty.

Technique

1   Shampoo, condition and blow dry client's hair.
2   Wrap set or cane row the hair using method described earlier in this chapter. Hair can be cane rowed in any fashion, whether it is circular, horizontal or diagonal, or can simply be cane rowed into one. The method is not important as the net will be covering the hair.
3   Place net over entire head (a).
4   Spray holding spray/spritz over entire head and use a blow dryer to seal the net in place (b).

5 Once dried, cut the outer perimeter of the net, following the shape of the client's head (c).

6 Using a razor, separate extension hair where it is sewn together to produce two weft strips (d).

7 Measure weft extensions horizontally to area of the head where the extensions are to be placed (e).

8 Apply bonding glue to weft strip or sew weft extensions to cane rowed base and net. Again, bear in mind the desired style to be achieved. If the hair is sparse in areas, sew weft to net only and continue until it is possible to sew weft to net and cane rowed base again (f).

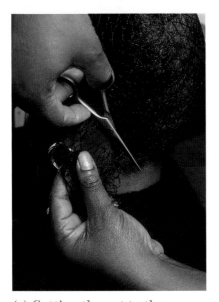

Before

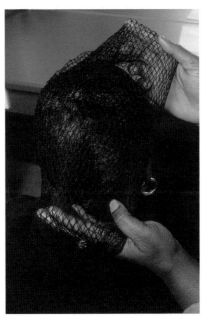

(a) Net placed on wrapped hair

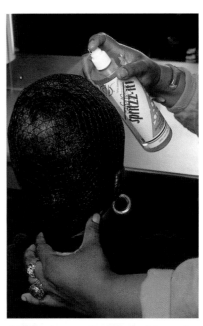

(b) Spritz applied to hold net in place

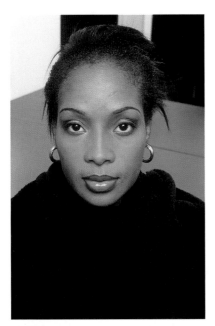

(c) Cutting the net to the contour of the head

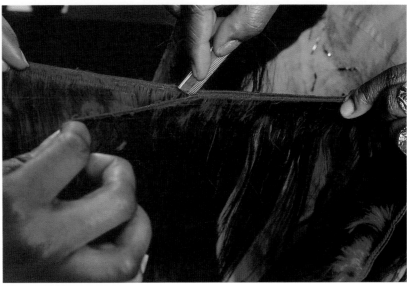

(d) Separating the wefts with a razor

9 Continue sewing/bonding, placing weft at measured spaces apart from each other. Do not place them too far apart otherwise the final look will be lacking in body.

10 Once the crown is reached, begin to place wefts in a circular fashion, working towards the centre of the head (g).

11 Once finished, cut a small bit of weft and use the end of a tail comb push this bit of weft in the centre so that no gaps are showing in the head (h).

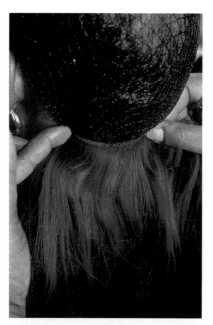

(e) Measuring weft

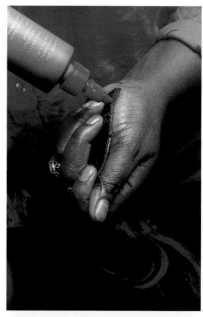

(f) Applying bonding glue

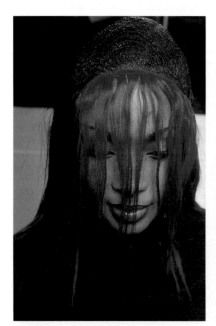

(g) Weft placed in circular fashion

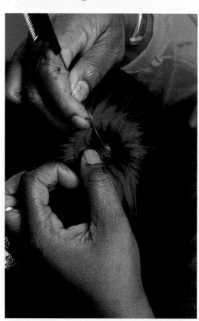

(h) Centre closure of weft

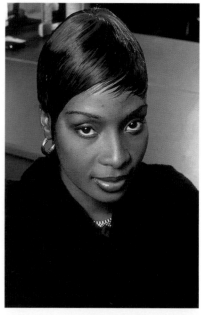

(i) Wrap set with wrap lotion

12 Apply wrapping lotion to entire head, wrap set and dry hair (i).

13 Once dried, cut and style as desired.

The finished style

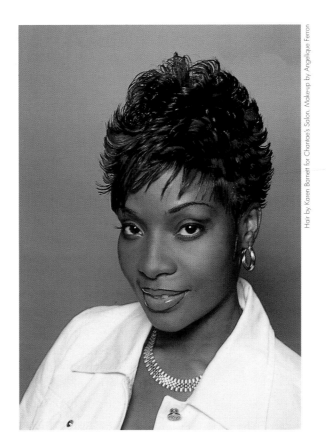

Hair by Karen Barnett for Chantae's Salon. Makeup by Angelique Ferron

Extensions using the cap technique

The cap technique is one where weft extensions are bonded to a soft mesh like material which fits snugly to the head like a cap. One of the advantages of this technique is that because the cap fits the contour of the head, the whole appearance is more natural. In addition, the cap can be removed and replaced as and when the client likes in the same way as a wig. This technique allows the user flexibility as well as a tailored look which meets the client's needs and is custom built for the individual. A further advantage is that if a client has long hair and would like a short look without having to cut her hair, the cap technique allows her the best of both worlds.

One of the disadvantages of using the cap technique, however, is that after a while the cap can shrink and become too small to fit the head as it should. This then means that the durability of this technique can be short and it can be expensive to keep repeating this process on an ongoing basis.

When carrying out the cap technique, the client's hair is normally wrap set so that it lies flat on the head. Cling film is then placed over the entire head followed by the cap. The cling film prevents the bonding glue from seeping through the mesh cap onto the client's hair.

Technique

1 Shampoo, condition and wrap set or cane row the client's hair (see Chapters 3 and 4) (a).
2 Place cling film over the entire head, keeping it as flat and as close to the head as possible (b).
3 Place cap over cling film and stretch it so that it fits snugly to the head (c).
4 Take the weft extension hair and, as for the mesh technique described above, use a razor or a pair of scissors to separate the two wefts which have been sewn together to produce one weft strip.
5 Using bonding glue, start bonding single wefts to the cap, cutting weft strips to fit across the head in accordance with the desired style to be achieved. Single wefts can be placed closer together so that it gives a more natural appearance.
6 Work upwards, placing wefts in line with the contour of the head (d).

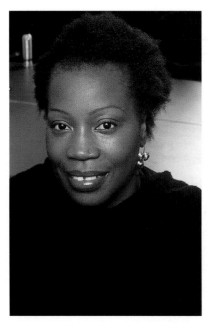 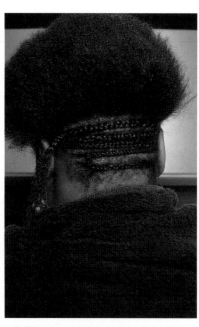 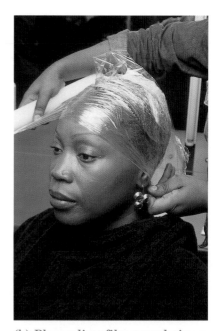

Before

(a) Cane rowing hair prior to cling film placement

(b) Place cling film over hair

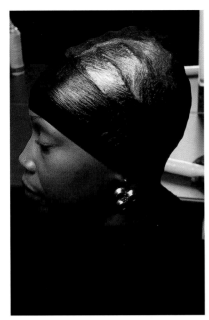

(c) Place cap over head

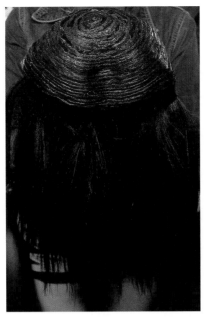

(d) Inside of cap weave showing spiral placement technique of weft

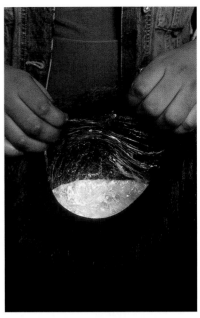

(e) Remove cling film

7   Follow steps 10–13 described on pages 242–5 for mesh technique.

8   Take off cap and remove cling film from the net and weft base (e).

9   Replace cap, cut and style weave.

The finished look

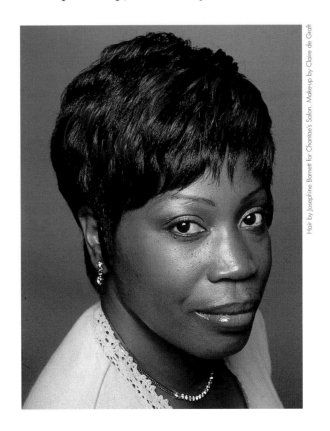

Hair by Josephine Barnett for Chantae's Salon. Make-up by Claire de Graft

Cutting and styling

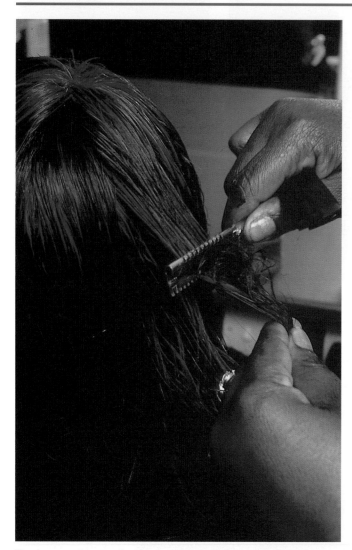

Razor cutting technique

The principles for cutting and styling extensions are the same as for cutting and styling the client's own hair. However, because extensions add bulk to the hair, it is sometimes necessary when cutting to thin out some of the hair. This can be achieved using a pair of thinning scissors or a razor.

If using synthetic hair for cane rowing or plaiting, it is advisable to choose a length which does not require cutting once completed. There may be some evening up of the ends to do, but a full hair cut should be avoided as it may distort the natural pattern in the hair and create an unnatural appearance.

As a general rule synthetic hair cannot be thermal styled as it is made up of nylon. However, some synthetic hair can withstand moderate heat and thermal styling is possible using warm, not hot hair curling irons.

Human hair, on the other hand, can be treated more like the client's own hair and because there are more styling options it can be blow-dried, thermal styled or set. Again, because weft hair can be slightly bulkier than natural hair, when human hair extensions are club cut it tends to look heavy on the ends, giving it an unnatural appearance. It may therefore be necessary to thin out some of the hair with thinning scissors or, for shorter looks, use a razor rather than scissors for cutting. The use of a razor takes bulk out of the weft hair and gives an overall softer feel to the hair cut. For more information on cutting see Chapter 10.

Note

All the hair used for hair extensions in this chapter was sponsored by Montaz of London.

Hair extensions equipment and maintenance table

Technique	Equipment	Aftercare	Shampoo	Conditioner	Removal
Cane row	Tail comb Section clips Hair for extensions	The scalp may become dry. Advise client to use oil sheen or braid spray as and when necessary.	If necessary, hair can be shampooed during the wearing of cane rows. Use cleansing shampoo first, then a moisturising shampoo to replace moisture. Use only gentle movements.	Liquid leave-in conditioner should be used as a cream conditioner may not rinse out fully.	Use a tail comb to separate the plaits at the end of the cane rows. Unpick cane rows and use a wide toothed comb to comb hair free. Shampoo and condition hair, preferably giving a deep penetrating treatment at this stage.
Single plaits	Tail comb Section clips Hair for extensions	A light scalp hairdress, oil sheen or braid spray can be applied as and when necessary.	Shampoo with care, concentrating on scalp area. If curly extensions have been used do not use vigorous movements during shampooing as this may cause the hair to tangle.	A cream or liquid moisturising conditioner can be used, but liquid conditioner will penetrate better. A cream conditioner may cause hair plaited with human hair to loosen.	Same as above. Note however, that after extensions have been removed and the client's hair is being combed, care must be taken because during the time of wearing the extensions there will be a build up of dirt and oils which would have collected at the base of the plait. This sometimes forms a knot and, if not combed out with care, can bring about excessive shedding.
Fashion locks using yarn/wool	Tail comb Section clips Yarn to be used for extensions	Initially braid spray or oil sheen can be used until new hair starts to grow through. The client should return to the salon every 2–3 months to have roots retwisted to	Hair can be shampooed as often as client wishes during the first 2–3 months before twisting begins to take place. A cleansing and moisturising shampoo should be used. Once twisting begins, the hair should be shampooed less often because this will make the twists unravel and	It would be better to use a liquid leave-in conditioner as the yarn is so dense that a cream conditioner will be of little or no effect.	Do not remove for at least six months if the intention is that the natural hair can begin to lock. Once this has taken place, the yarn extensions can be cut off gradually or completely.

Hair extensions equipment and maintenance table

Technique	Equipment	Aftercare	Shampoo	Conditioner	Removal
Fashion locks using yarn/wool (continued)		start forming locks to the natural hair. At this time oil sheen or a hairdress alone should be used; any liquid spray will cause the twists to unravel.	the hair will then have to be retwisted.		
Sewn weave	Tail comb Denman brush Section clips Thread Thread cutter Weave needle (preferably curved) Razor/thinning scissors	Use oil sheen or a light hair oil applied directly to the scalp. Avoid the use of braid spray as this may affect the styling of the extension hair if it becomes too saturated with braid spray. Hair should be combed free of tangles daily and hair can be thermal styled as often as client desires depending on whether synthetic or human hair was used.	Hair should be combed free of tangles before shampooing. Section hair into four and plait each section. Follow manufacturer's instructions for shampooing.	Follow manufacturer's instructions. Alternatively use a light conditioner to assist the combing out of any tangles.	Starting from the nape comb hair free of tangles, then using a thread cutter or a pair of scissors, carefully cut thread used for sewing. Care must be taken not to cut the client's own hair during this process. Undo cane rowed base, comb hair with a wide toothed comb then shampoo and condition with a deep penetrating conditioner.

Hair extensions equipment and maintenance table

Technique	Equipment	Aftercare	Shampoo	Conditioner	Removal
Bonding	Tail comb Section clips Denman brush Razor if necessary Weft hair Bonding glue Glue solvent Razor/thinning scissors	Avoid applying too much force during combing/brushing as this could put too much stress on the client's natural hair. Avoid using a lot of hair oil as this could loosen the bonding. Hair can be thermal styled as often as client desires.	Comb hair with a wide toothed comb or brush hair to remove tangles. Shampoo with care as this could loosen bonding. Use cleansing shampoo. Where bonding has become detached, re-apply bonding glue after shampooing.	Avoid using cream conditioners as this could loosen bonding. A liquid conditioner is suitable.	Comb/brush hair free of tangles. Apply bonding remover/glue solvent to root area of each section. Do this to the entire head so as to allow the areas applied first to soften. Starting at one end of the weft, lift it away from the client's hair. This should peel away easily. If not, apply more remover or, alternatively, apply a heavy cream conditioner to the root area and place client under a warm dryer. Once removed, comb hair carefully as some of the glue may still be left on the hair. If care is not taken, hair breakage may occur.
Laser weave	Tail comb Section clips Hair for extensions Laser gun Glue sticks Glue solvent Denman brush Razor/thinning scissors	Hair can be treated as client's own hair. Oil sheen, hair sprays, scalp hairdress can all be used. However, care must be taken when combing/brushing – start	Hair can be shampooed as if it is client's own hair. A cleansing and moisturising shampoo should be used. Hair can be roller set or blow-dried with a round brush.		A hair-friendly solvent should be used to dissolve the glue. Once all extensions have been removed, shampoo and condition hair giving the client a deep penetrating hair treatment at this stage. Extensions can either be replaced or discarded.

Hair extensions equipment and maintenance table

Technique	Equipment	Aftercare	Shampoo	Conditioner	Removal
Laser weave (continued)		from the ends of the hair and work towards the root.			Depending on whether the stitched or bonding method has been used, follow the appropriate removal technique as described above.
Mesh technique	Tail comb Section clips Holding spray Denman brush Hair net Weft hair Depending on technique, thread and curved needle for stitching or glue for bonding. Razor/thinning scissor	Use oil sheen. Avoid using too much holding spray as this will filter through net to the hair underneath and cause build up.	Although it is possible to shampoo this type of weave, it is advisable not to as it will be impossible to shampoo the scalp area properly due to the fact that the net is placed between the client's hair and the weft hair. If the stitched method is used then shampooing is easier. If the bonding method is used, advise client not to shampoo but remove weave after 2–3 weeks. If shampooing is absolutely necessary, then shampoo with care using a cleansing and a mositurising shampoo.	If the hair has been shampooed, use either a liquid leave-in conditioner or a light cream conditioner to detangle	
Cap technique 'The Wig'	Tail comb Section clips Hair spray Wrapping lotion/ oil moisturiser for wrapping hair prior to cutting. Denman brush Razor/thinning scissors.	As this technique is similar to a 'wig' effect, it can be removed and replaced as and when the client desires. Once removed, it can be placed on a wig stand to	Do not apply vigorous movements whilst shampooing, use gentle squeezing actions. Use cleansing shampoo.	Light conditioner to be used. After shampooing and conditioning, check hair for any loosening of bonding and reapply if necessary or remove weft strip	The cap weave simply needs to be discarded after use.

Hair extensions equipment and maintenance table

Technique	Equipment	Aftercare	Shampoo	Conditioner	Removal
Cap technique 'The Wig' (continued)	Cling film Weave cap Bonding glue Weft hair	maintain shape. It can be thermal styled as often as the client desires.		and apply a new strip.	

Natural hair

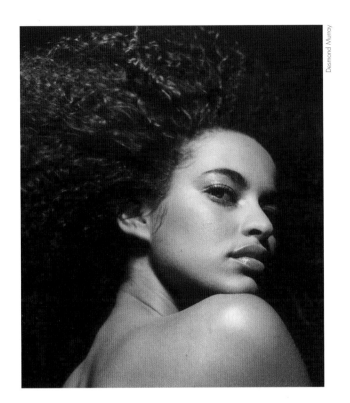

Desmond Murray

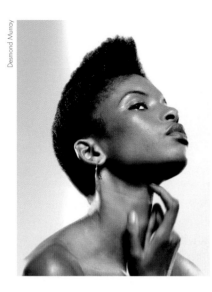

Desmond Murray

For years, Africans have plaited their natural hair into intricate styles using adornments and extensions such as vegetable fibres, wool or sometimes the hair from relatives who have cut their hair, to add to the intricacy of the style. Very often, styles were designed to depict special occasions such as births, deaths, marriage, coming of age and cultural events.

Early accounts of styling black hair, post slavery, seem to come from America. Otherwise, very little seems to be documented on black people's experiences with hair in England and the Caribbean. What is known, however, is that product development started in America with tools such as pressing combs and later on products such as relaxers. These, however, were crude and basic and often led to extreme hair and scalp damage.

Although such early items came as a breakthrough in the black haircare market, it was often felt that the use of chemicals and the pressing of naturally curly hair was done to imitate styles worn by Caucasians. The late 1960s saw a radical change in the political stance of a number of African Americans and the black Civil Rights Movement was born. The political ethos of the movement was 'I'm black and proud': this brought with it a black consciousness which had a direct bearing on the black hair care industry and thus saw the emergence of the 'Afro' hairstyle, sometimes called the natural look.

The Afro was considered a militant style and was initially worn by political activists such as Angela Davis and Stokeley Carmichael. The Afro and all it stood for made the bold statement that black people were proud to wear their hair in its natural curly state.

It gained in popularity as actors, actresses and models sported this new look, and by the 1970s had become a mainstream fashion statement also worn by some Caucasians. During this period, the Afro transformed into Afro puffs with zig zag partings, asymetric cuts, block colouring and eventually the short Afro sculptured cut.

One of the offspills of the black movement was the increased awareness of Rastafarianism, which had its roots in religion and also brought with it the 'dreadlocks' style. Dreadlocks first came to prominence in the 1970s, however, a study of ancient African civilisation will reveal that hair locking, as with most natural hairstyles today, is not a new technique.

The dreadlocks of the 1970s devised its rationale from the biblical figure of Samson, who did not cut his hair but allowed it to grow in long locks. The grooming and cultivation of locks was deemed as sacred to the religious beliefs of the Rastafarian movement.

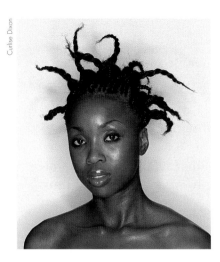

Curlise Dixon

As black people began to feel more comfortable with wearing their hair in its natural state, other hairstyles which were hitherto only worn indoors or worn by children were brought to the forefront of Afro hair styling. These styles included cane rowing and plaiting.

By the 1980s with the birth of the Gheri Curl natural hairstyles became less popular and throughout the 1980s and up to the mid 1990s, Gheri curls and relaxers took the lead as tools, products and aftercare treatments became more sophisticated, professional and less damaging to the hair. This change to chemically processing hair again did not mean that African-Americans or African-Caribbeans were no longer 'proud to be black', it simply afforded them another styling option, as styles and fashion changed they changed with it.

As fashions come and go and are repeated, there has been a new move over the last 10 years, back to the natural look. This has come about because of a worldwide move to re-educate people about the benefits of natural products, whether it be for food, medicine, beauty or hair products.

As people have been encouraged to question the type of cosmetics they buy, the type of foodstuffs they eat and drink, so they are being asked to consider why they are opting for chemically processing their hair rather than wearing their hair natural. The manufacturers of hair and beauty products have tapped into the natural market by using real plant extracts for their products rather than a synthetic formula. Thus, with an abundance of natural hair care products on the market, more and more people are making a conscious decision to wear their hair in its natural state or opt for fashion dreadlocks.

The styling of natural hair is now diverse, it can be left as a natural Afro, cane rowed, plaited, twisted, woven, dreadlocked, coloured or thermal styled/pressed for variety. All of these techniques are discussed in this chapter. Some of these looks, which once would not have been worn in public, have now become more widely acceptable and desirable. It is not surprising that specialist salons catering for natural hair have emerged and mainstream salons have had to take the increasing number of natural hair clients seriously by catering for their needs.

Consultation and analysis

Before carrying out any work on natural hair, it is necessary to conduct a consultation and analysis of the hair and scalp. Some of the more common problems noted when working with natural hair are:

- split ends
- dryness of hair
- dry scalp
- the use of dressings which are not easily absorbed by the hair or scalp
- styling and controlling hair in its naturally curly state
- and how to work with a client who is changing over from chemical processing to wearing natural hair.

Carrying out consultation and analysis

Follow the same procedure for consultation and analysis as described in Chapter 1. The following points should also be noted.

1   Unless the hair is worn in locks, use a wide-toothed comb and comb the hair carefully as natural hair has a tendency to tangle easily.
2   Check the hair for any split ends or hairline damage – otherwise known as traction alopecia – which can occur with natural hair which has been braided/plaited over long periods. Also check the hair for breakage where the hair has become too brittle or where there are two different textures on the shaft of the hair, i.e. where the client is growing out a chemical process and there is both natural hair and chemically processed hair along the hair shaft.

If the client attends the salon wearing braids/plaits and has asked for them to be removed and the natural hair to be shampooed and conditioned, extra care has to be taken when combing hair once plaits have been removed as the scalp could be quite tender at this stage. In addition, a build up of dirt and oils may have collected at the base of the plait forming a knot. This knot must be loosened carefully to avoid breakage and hair loss. It is worth noting here that when combing hair, some shedding will take place. This is simply because the hair has not been combed for a while and hair which would naturally have shed over the course of the wearing of plaits would now be coming away.

Shampooing and conditioning

As mentioned above, one of the problems encountered with natural hair is its tendency to become dry. In order to

Tip

Be sure to handle wet hair with care as, once wet, natural hair springs back to its natural curl pattern and this could range from wavy to excessively curly. The more tightly curled the hair is, the more susceptible it is to breakage if not handled correctly.

combat this, clients tend to overcompensate by applying what may appear to be too much maintenance product on the hair. This results in either a very oily or sticky feel and tends to attract more dirt particles to the hair.

The shampooing process therefore needs to thoroughly cleanse the hair to remove the maintenance product. If any remains, it can affect styling processes such as blow-drying/pressing and the hair will have a tendency to smell unpleasant and emit smoke during the blow drying/pressing process.

There are many shampoos and conditioners on the market, and the resurgence of the natural hair look has brought about a host of new products. Some manufacturers use words such as 'natural', 'organic' and 'herbal' to describe hair maintenance preparations which boast of natural ingredients. As African-Caribbean hair has a tendency to be dry, it is necessary when working with natural hair to use a good moisture balanced shampoo and conditioner.

When shampooing natural hair, especially locks, avoid excessive agitation as this may cause the hair to tangle, or could tear the locks in the root area. Otherwise, see the maintenance table at the end of this chapter along with shampooing and conditioning techniques described in Chapter 3.

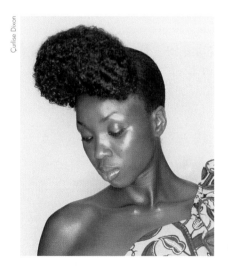

Curlise Dixon

Blow-drying natural hair

Blow-drying the hair helps to make it more pliable for styling and also stretches the natural hair, allowing the stylist, when working with short natural hair, to have a bit more length to work with, especially when braiding. Some styles such as twists do not require the hair to be blow-dried prior to styling, as drying of the hair is carried out after the twists are done. For further information on blowdrying see Chapter 5.

Use of hair oils/dressings

After blow-drying, the hair and scalp can be treated with hair oils/dressings. A hair oil/dressing should effectively moisturise the hair and scalp, making the hair more pliable to work with. It should not be too heavy as this will only attract more dirt to the hair. Hair oil/dressings can be applied directly to the scalp and the hair; be careful not to use too much product. The hair is now ready for cane rowing, braiding, twisting, weaving, thermal styling or natural styling as the client desires.

Cane row

Tip

For aftercare, shampooing, conditioning and removal see the maintenance table at the end of Chapter 12.

This style is ideal for natural hair as it can be worn with or without extensions.

The life span of cane rows (without extensions) is not very long and can last from 1 to 4 weeks, depending on the length of hair. Ideally cane rows should not be kept for more than two weeks as the hair begins to look untidy after this. The removal of this type of cane rows is usually an easy process. This however will depend on the thickness and the number of cane rows carried out. The smaller the cane rows, the longer it will take to remove them. It is not uncommon to see some shedding of the hair at this stage. This is because the hair would not have been combed for several days/weeks and it is hair which would have been lost naturally through daily combing.

Technique

- Follow technique for cane rowing as described in Chapter 12 except that it is done without extensions.

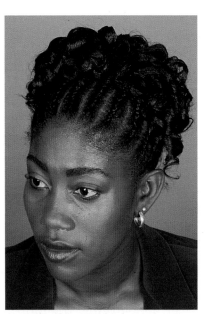 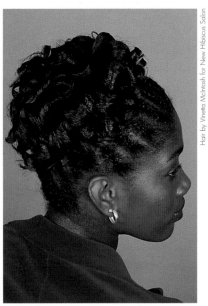

Finished plaits – front

Finished plaits – side

French plait

A French plait can be created by using the same technique to braid the hair in a single plait from the crown to the nape.

Technique

1 Brush the hair to remove all tangles.

2 With the head tilted backwards, divide the foremost hair into three equal sections (a).

3 Starting from either the left or the right, cross an outside strand over the centre strand. Repeat this action with the opposite outer strand (b).

4 Section a fourth strand (less in thickness than the initial three strands) and incorporate this with an outside strand (c).

5 Cross the thickened strand over the centre, and repeat this step with the opposite outer strand (d).

6 Continue this sequence of adding hair to the outer strand, before crossing it over the centre (e).

7 When there is no more hair to be added, continue plaiting down to the ends and secure them (f).

Variety can be added to the finished plait by plaiting the hair underneath. This is the reverse of the technique described above and will cause the finished plait to be raised.

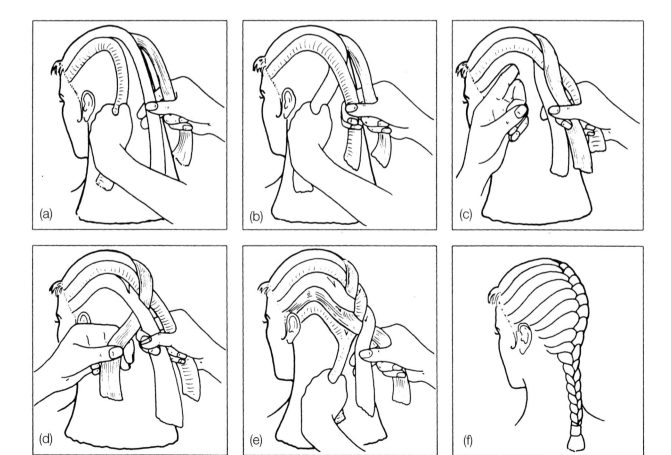

A three-stem (head-hugging) plait

Single plaiting

For years Africans have plaited their natural hair into intricate hairstyles, which very often evolved from and related to special events in their life. Hairstyles were designed and styled to mark special occasions such as births, deaths, marriages, coming of age and cultural events. Single plaiting without extensions is an old technique for grooming hair, not only for people of African descent but across most cultures. The single plaiting technique could involve the designing of a new hairstyle with lots of plaits or only a few.

When natural hair is plaited without extensions, the plaits can last for anything from one day to several weeks depending on the length of the hair. On longer hair the plaits may last for quite a while, but they will begin to look shabby after about two weeks so it is advisable not to leave them in for longer than that. Removing this type of single plait is less time consuming than those using hair extensions.

Tip

For aftercare, shampooing, conditioning and removal see the maintenance table at the end of this chapter.

Technique

- Follow the technique for single plaiting as described on page 223 but without using extensions.

Zulu knots

Tip

As an alternative, the hair can be twisted and then knotted and secured with a pin or clip.

Zulu knots come from the South African Zulu people. The hair can either be twisted or plaited and then twisted round itself to form a tight coil or knot. Today, zulu knots are worn as a fun style with an avant-garde feel to it. The style is suitable for relaxed or natural hair or dreadlocks. The hair can be divided into squares or asymmetric shapes to create variety and individual flair.

Technique

Prepare the hair according to the hair type and style requirements. (For further information see Chapters 3 and 5.) Select a suitable dressing or oil sheen spray depending on the hair type as discussed previously.

Equipment needed:

- Denman brush
- de-tangling comb
- tail comb.

1 Gown the client.

2 Comb the hair through thoroughly and section the hair as required.

3 Take a section of hair and plait it from roots to ends (a).

4 Wrap the plait in a circular fashion, working from the roots to the ends (b).

5 Tuck the ends under the plait and secure with a bent pin or a grip (c).

6 Continue sectioning, plaiting and twisting the hair until the whole head is complete.

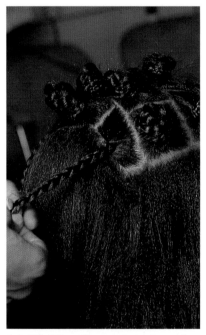

(a) Plaiting from roots to ends

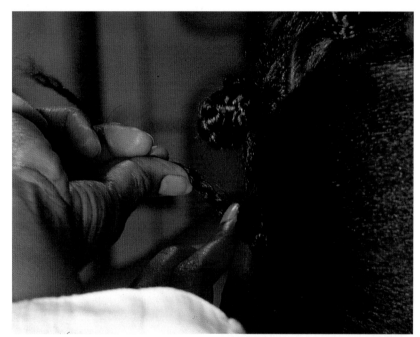

(b) Creating the knot

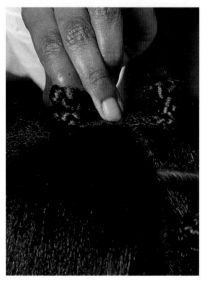

(c) Securing the ends

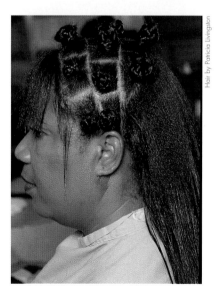

Half head of Zulu knots

Hair by Patricia Livingston

Single twists

Single and double twists help to keep natural hair neat and well groomed. They have become more popular as clients still wanting to maintain their natural hair sought an alternative to braided styles. Twists can be kept for up to one month before the style begins to look untidy. Hair that is short and coarse in texture is unlikely to last as long as one month. However, because no chemical product is used, hair can be shampooed, conditioned and retwisted as often as necessary.

Twists are usually carried out using a pomade or a gel and pomade combination; some manufacturers have products specifically designed for natural hair. When using a gel and pomade mixture, the gel ensures that the style can be maintained for at least a couple of weeks and the pomade provides sheen and prevents the hair from drying out with the use of the gel.

Technique

1   Shampoo, condition, towel dry and section hair into four.
2   Using the tail comb, section the hair horizontally, starting at the nape of the head. Keep rest of the hair out of the way using section clips or butterfly clips.

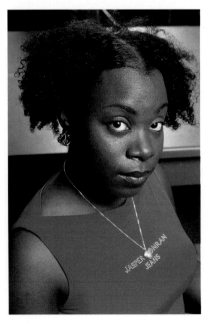

Before

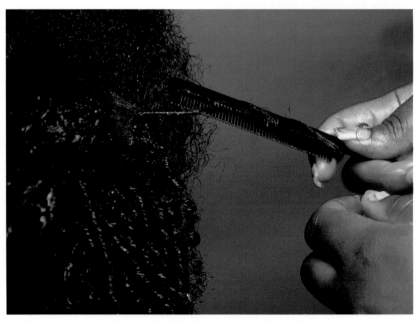

(a) Using the comb to twist the hair starting at the roots

Tip

When using a mixture of styling gel and pomade to twist hair, ensure that the mixture consists more of pomade than styling gel as too much styling gel may ultimately make the hair feel dry and harsh over a long period.

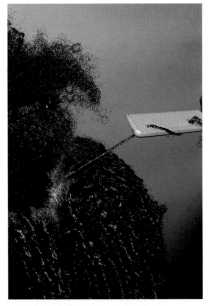 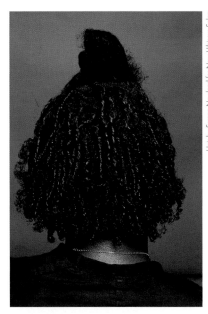

Hair by Serena Newland for New Hibiscus Salon

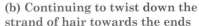
(b) Continuing to twist down the strand of hair towards the ends   **Completed twists**

3   Divide horizontal sections into sub-sections which should be about $\frac{1}{8}$ inch in diameter for effective twisting.

4   Apply product for twisting to entire length of hair.

5   Using the tail comb, start twisting the hair from the root by placing the comb close to the root and rotating it clockwise, sliding down the hair with each rotation until the end is reached (a).

6   Continue working up the head, taking diagonal sections and placing each twist in brick formation so as to avoid gaps appearing in the hair style (b).

7   Once all the hair has been twisted, arrange twists neatly in the direction in which it should fall, then place the client under a warm dryer to dry the hair. This process usually takes about 20–40 minutes depending on hair texture and thickness of each twisted section.

8   Once completely dried, spray hair with a sheen spray.

If the client intends to grow locks from twisting, the stylist must advise the client to return to the salon every 6–8 weeks to have the hair retwisted until locks are formed.

Tip

For aftercare, shampooing, conditioning and removal see the maintenance table at the end of this chapter.

Double twists

Double twists employ the same technique as single twists except that each section is subdivided into two strands which are then wrapped around each other.

Technique

1 Follow the same procedure for single twist up to step 4.

2 Instead of using a tail comb, divide the subsection into two and, using fingers, twist one section over the other in a clockwise fashion, always taking the left section of hair and twisting it over the right section.

3 Continue working up the head in a brick formation until all double twists are completed.

4 Continue as for single twists steps 8 and 9.

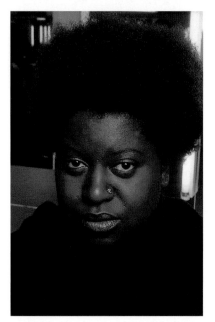

Before

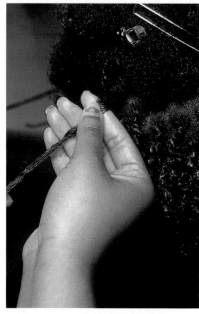

Apply product to the hair

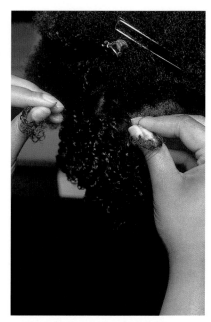

Divide hair into two sections and twist around each other

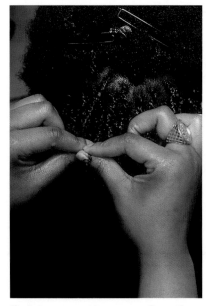

Twist one section over the other

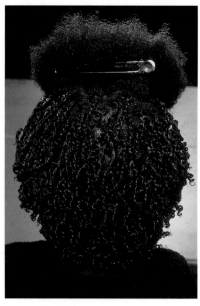

Completed back

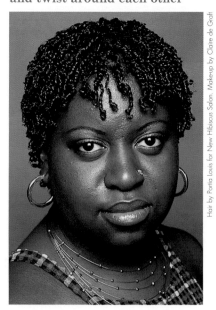

Double twists – finished look

Hair by Portia Louis for New Hibiscus Salon. Makeup by Claire de Graft

Senegalese/root twists

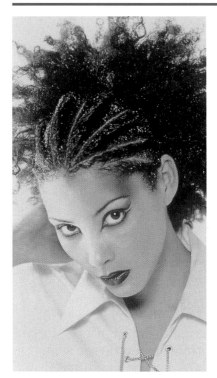

Traditional Senegalese twist

As the name suggests, this style has its origins in the West African state of Senegal and can be used to create intricate patterns on natural hair or chemically processed hair. Today it is created using styling gel or a mixture of styling gel and hair pomade which is used for creating single and double twists. It can be carried out using the fingers or a tail comb. The photo below shows the twists being created using the fingers. When the twists are completed, the ends of the hair can be maintained by either setting or using curling irons to create curl clusters and add variety to the style. The method described is non traditional and creates Senegalese twists in a criss-cross fashion.

Technique

1 Before twisting, carry out a consultation and analysis to ascertain the desired style.

2 The hair should then be shampooed, conditioned and blow-dried in preparation. Blow-drying natural hair prior to Senegalese twisting helps to control the hair. The hair can be pressed for a straighter look.

3 Once a desired style is chosen begin to map out sections of hair for twisting (a).

4 Using fingers, start close to the root, taking a small section of hair and twisting it in a clockwise fashion (b).

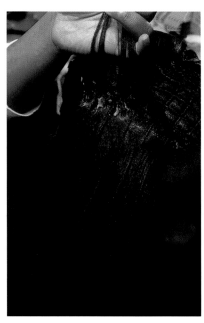

(a) Mapping out sections

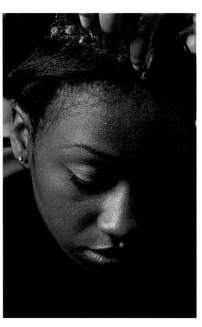

(b) Starting twist technique at the root front hairline

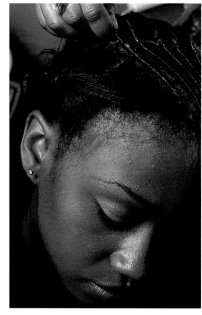

Completed Senegalese twists

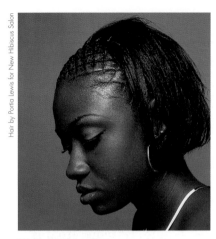

Finished look

Work along the channel, taking up more sections of hair as the twists form.

5   When one channel is finished, a band can be used to hold hair in place until all twists are completed.

6   At this stage, the ends of the hair can be single/double twisted or the client may opt for the ends to be thermal styled with curling irons. If the ends are to be thermal styled, first place the client under a dryer to dry twists in place.

7   Once dried, the ends of the hair can now be styled as desired.

8   Spray a sheen spray over entire head to keep hair pliable.

Dreadlocks

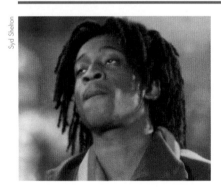

The decision to lock hair is one which should be given a great deal of consideration. Once the locking process has taken place, there is no turning back and any change of heart will result in the client having to cut off all the locked hair and start afresh. Adequate time should be set aside during consultation and analysis to discuss the different locking processes, the length of time it would take before the hair begins to lock and the maintenance of hair before and after the locking stages. Once a decision is made then the stylist can proceed with the locking process of the client's choice.

The photo opposite (locks before root retwist) shows locks which were started off with the yarn method (see Chapter 12 on hair extensions for technique and more information). These extensions were gradually cut as the hair grew and twisting began. Locking took place over a period of six months.

Locks Retwist

Technique

1   Gown and towel client.

2   Starting at the nape, separate locks by easing them apart from each other in the root area. If separation has been done regularly, there should be minimum matting in the root area (a).

3   Once all separation has been carried out, shampoo and condition hair using the appropriate shampoo and conditioner (see the maintenance table at the end of this chapter).

4 Towel blot hair, apply spray-on leave-in conditioner and place client under a warm dryer to remove excess water.

5 Begin retwisting starting at the nape and using product of your choice. In this instance, a mixture of styling gel and pomade is used. Keep the rest of the hair out of the way using section clips.

6 Twist hair from the root using a clockwise twisting technique. The tension should be even and not too tight as this could cause breakage in the root area. Apply enough product so that as twist is worked along the length of the lock, any hair which may have become detached from the lock can be worked back into the locks (b) & (c).

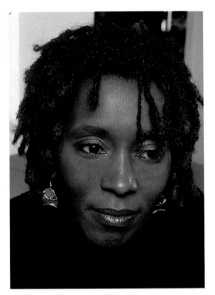

Locks before root retwist

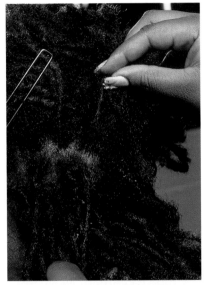

(a) Separating locks at the root

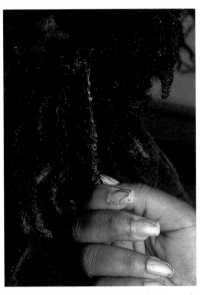

(c) Twisting lock through to ends

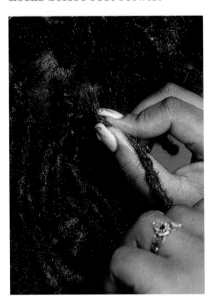

(b) Applying product and starting twist at roots

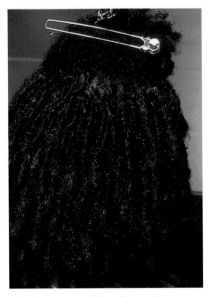

(d) Completed back section

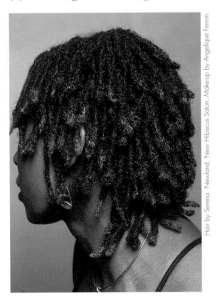

Finished look

Hair by Serena Newland, New Hibiscus Salon. Makeup by Angelique Ferron.

7   Continue working up the head until all locks are retwisted (d).

8   Place client under a warm dryer until all of the new twists and locks are dried.

9   Spray oil sheen over entire head.

Any other options?

One of the problems that the wearers of natural hair face is the lack of versatility when styling. It is probably the one factor that propels those with natural hair into chemically processing their hair. There are a couple of options available:

1   Adding colour to the hair in the form of tints or bleach.

2   As a temporary measure, hair can be thermally styled, which is more commonly known as pressing.

Addition of colour

Colour added to natural hair does help to bring it alive. Whilst this can be done quite safely because there are no other chemicals on the hair, there is one pitfall which is that it tends to make hair which has a tendency to be dry even drier.

If colouring/bleaching is favoured by a client, mix a few drops of oil into the tint or bleach before application to lessen the harsh effect of colourant/bleach and avoid drying out hair too much. Most product manufacturers will have an oil based product specifically designed to work in this way.

For the colouring process and more information on colouring see Chapter 11.

Tip

When bleaching locks, it will be necessary to carry out several applications in order to achieve the desired colour, due to the density of the locks.

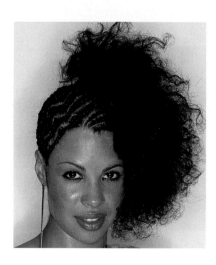 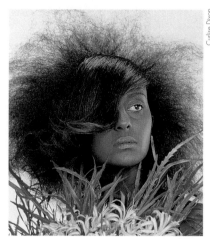

Curlise Dixon

Styling options

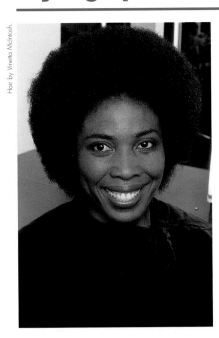

Hair by Vinetta McIntosh.

As discussed earlier, the art of pressing, as it is known today, dates back to the early 1900s. Prior to this, there was a very crude method using knives or forks which were heated over open fires then applied to the hair in order to stretch it.

Pressing, along with curling, became increasingly popular and rose to its pinnacle in the 1960s. Since then the press and curl market has slowed down with the advent of more professional products for chemically straightening and perming hair. However, with the present increase in natural hair treatment, there has been a noticeable rise in the demand for press and curl in salons, along with other fashion looks such as partial pressing (see also Chapter 9 for more information on thermal styling/pressing).

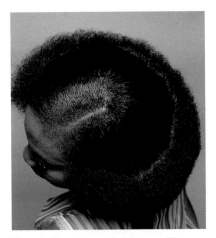
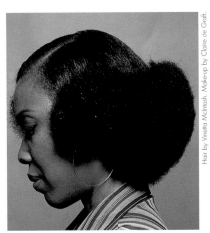

Hair by Vinetta McIntosh. Makeup by Claire de Graft.

Partially pressed Afro puff

A change from chemically processed hair to natural hair

Finally, what can be done for the client who has a relaxer or perm and now wants to go natural? How does one work with hair which is partially natural and partially chemically processed?

The decision to change from chemical processing to natural styling is a major one and it should be discussed in depth with the client. The options available are:

- waiting until sufficient new hair grows and cutting off all existing chemically processed hair

- plaiting or cane rowing hair until sufficient new growth

- weaving hair with or without extensions whilst gradually cutting off processed hair

- simply shampooing and conditioning hair, again gradually cutting processed ends until only the natural hair remains.

In most cases, if the client's hair is already short, there may be little or no objection to cutting off all of the existing chemically processed hair. However, it is more difficult if the hair is long and the client does not want to lose too much of the length. As mentioned above, one of the options is to wear the hair in extensions until there is sufficient new hair for the client to feel comfortable with wearing their own hair natural.

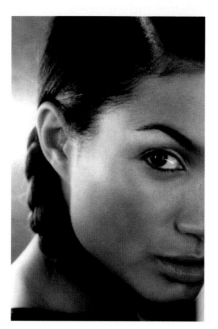 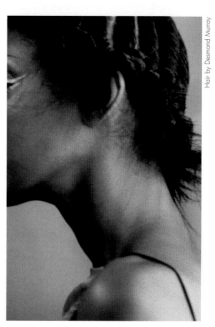

Hair by Desmond Murray

If the client does not opt for extensions but wishes to allow the natural hair to grow through whilst the rest of the hair remains processed, this can pose problems for both the stylist and the client. The two different textures of hair can cause uneven tension and the hair can begin to shed at the point where the natural hair meets with the processed hair.

If the client's natural hair is of a soft/wavy texture, there may be minimum breakage because the two textures may not be acutely different. As an alternative, but only a temporary measure, any natural hair present can be thermal styled/pressed to even out texture. This should not be done often and only carried out with extreme caution, taking care not to overlap too much into the processed hair with the pressing comb as, over a period of time, this will cause too much stress to the processed hair.

Clients who opt to wait until there is sufficient new growth whilst keeping the hair that is already processed sometimes become tired with the waiting process and, more often than not, opt for chemical processing again. It is the duty of the stylist to have another consultation with the client and to make alternative suggestions.

The best option usually is to advise the client to put the hair in extensions, allowing the new hair to grow through and not putting too much stress on the processed hair. The client can decide when the natural hair is at a length where she feels comfortable about cutting off all the processed hair. She must be advised against the constant use of hair extensions as this may cause hairline damage.

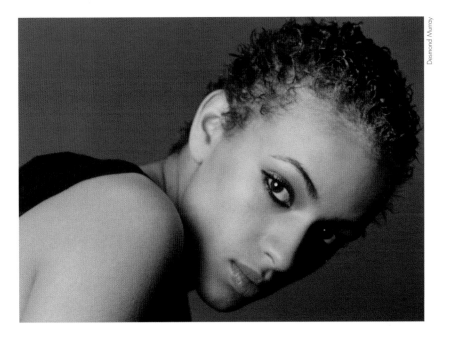

Desmond Murray

Natural haircare equipment and maintenance table

Technique	Equipment	Aftercare	Shampoo	Conditioner	Removal
Cane row, single plaits and Zulu knots	Detangling comb Tail comb Section clips	Spray with oil sheen or apply light hair oil to the scalp. Do not use liquid braid spray because of added water which would revert hair which was previously blow-dried or thermal pressed.	As this sytle is done fairly often, shampooing usually takes place once the plaits or knots have been removed. However, if client wishes to shampoo whilst wearing the style, use gentle movements. Use a cleansing then a moisturising shampoo.	Use a liquid leave-in conditioner Avoid using cream conditioners as it may not be rinsed out fully and therefore becomes trapped between styled hair. After conditioning, place client under a warm drier.	Use a metal end tail comb to loosen end of the plait if necessary. Use a larger comb to comb through the rest of the hair until all plaits/knots have been removed. A deep penetrating treatment should be given at this stage. If hair is styled in Zulu knots, first take out pins which are holding knots in place, unwind knots and undo plaits.
Single/double/Senegalese twists	Same as above plus: product for twisting – gel and pomade mixture or manufacturer's own brand designed specifically for natural hair.	Use oil sheen/light hair oil/dressing. No liquid sprays should be used as this will loosen twists.	Unless twists are to be removed, shampooing should be avoided as this will loosen the twists.	To be avoided unless twists are removed completely.	Dampen hair first to loosen gel used for twisting. With Senegalese twists, cut bands used to keep hair in place using a pair of regular scissors and taking care not to cut the client's hair. Comb hair with a wide-toothed comb and proceed to shampoo and condition. A deep penetrating treatment should be given at this stage.
Dreadlocks	Same as above unless client prefers to use	Same as above except that client will need to	Shampooing should take place only when hair has	Use a liquid leave-in conditioner.	Once locking has taken place, the only way to remove locks is to cut them off. If locking

Natural haircare equipment and maintenance table

Technique	Equipment	Aftercare	Shampoo	Conditioner	Removal
	yarn extensions for a dreadlocks effect. If this is the case, see Chapter 12 on hair extensions for more information.	return to the salon every 6–8 weeks to re-twist the root area.	begun to lock. Use a cleansing shampoo, then a moisturising shampoo.		hasn't started taking place see removal technique for twists above,

Black skin care and make-up

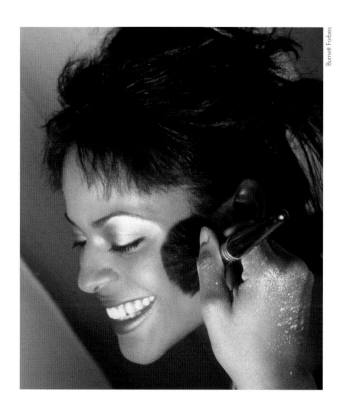

14

Burnett Forbes

Learning objectives

This chapter covers the following:

- **the structure of the skin**
- **skin types**
- **differences between African-Caribbean and Caucasian skin**
- **skin disorders**
- **analysis**
- **skin care and cosmetics**
- **make-up techniques**

Skin types

Tip

Never assume that an African-Caribbean skin is necessarily oily. Automatically treating skin that is normal or dry as an oily skin can lead to dehydration, which then leads to hyper-pigmentation – the accumulation of pigment in an area resulting in darker patches and uneven skin tone.

Characteristics of African-Caribbean skin

Due to the characteristics of African-Caribbean skin it would appear to identify with a particular skin type, namely an oily skin. However, it would be incorrect to assume that because the skin is African-Caribbean it is oily. Each person that enters the salon should be treated as an individual and a skin analysis/diagnosis is required for all clients. (See Chapter 2 for information on the structure of the skin.)

African-Caribbean skins:

- tend to be oily due to their greater number of sebaceous glands and may suffer with comodones (blackheads) and spots
- tend to suffer uneven pigmentation. (Following trauma to the skin such as spots, cuts and grazes, pigments rush to the affected area to aid the healing process and therefore leave the area darker.)
- tend to flake due to the skin desquamating (shedding) frequently – hyper-keratosis, the overgrowth of the horny layer (see page 295). When African-Caribbean skins desquamate, there is a tendency for them to have an ashy or greyish appearance. To help counteract this, in addition to professional attention, a good home-care routine is advised including the use of a facial scrub which will aid the removal of the dead skin cells
- tend to dehydrate due to the frequency of the skin desquamating. When skin sheds at the rate of African-Caribbean skin it tends to dry out and lack natural moisture, therefore becoming dehydrated.

There are four main skin types: normal, dry, greasy and combination. Each type has its individual characteristics that makes it identifiable.

Normal skin

- balanced skin type associated with young skin
- even oil secretion, not too oily or too dry
- generally blemish free with even pigmentation
- smooth, soft, supple skin surface
- healthy glow

- medium thickness of epidermis and firm to touch
- high degree of elasticity
- pores are medium to small.

Dry skin

- dry to the touch with a rough, coarse texture
- under-active sebaceous glands and poor moisture content
- tendency to have broken capillaries, milia (around eyes and cheeks), freckles and uneven pigmentation
- premature wrinkling starting around the eyes
- dull, pale appearance
- thin epidermis
- feels tight after washing
- pores are small to tight
- tendency to flaky patches
- prone to sensitivity.

Greasy skin

- oily due to over-active sebaceous glands (may be hormonal)
- prone to comodones, pustules and uneven pigmentation
- wrinkling not apparent until later years due to high degree of elasticity
- sallow complexion due to the build-up of dead skin cells and excess sebum clogging the pores
- thick epidermis
- enlarged pore size caused by the high rate of oil secretion
- high moisture content.

Combination skin

This skin type has characteristics from two or more of the other main skin types. Usually a combination skin is part dry and part greasy. The dry areas of the face tend to be the eyes and cheeks, with the oilier skin being on the forehead and centre panel (nose and chin) commonly known as the 'T zone'.

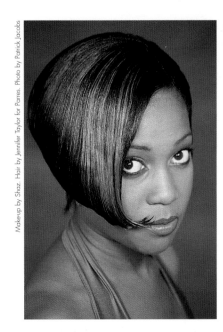

Makeup by Shaz. Hair by Jennifer Taylor for Parres. Photo by Patrick Jacobs

Tip

When removing make-up it may be necessary to re-apply cleanser until all the make-up is removed before carrying out the toning process.

Skin care

A skin care routine is essential for all skin types. It is necessary to cleanse, tone and moisturise twice a day to maintain a healthy, well-nourished skin.

- **Cleansing** removes make-up, dirt and the top layers of dead skin cells whilst helping to relax and unblock pores. The eyes should be cleansed first using damp cotton wool and eye make-up remover, working from the outer corner of the eye and under the lower lashes to the inner corner of the eye and over the eye lid, using gentle sweeping and circular movements. Wipe over again with clean, damp cotton wool. Next the lips. Place two fingers at the corner of the mouth to provide support. Using damp cotton wool and cleanser, wipe across the lower and then upper lip. Incorporate gentle circular movements to help remove stubborn lipstick. Finally the face is cleansed. Apply cleanser onto the back of your non-working hand and then transfer it to your palms. Apply to the neck, chin, cheeks, nose and forehead using effleurage (stroking movements). Massage gently over the skin with your finger tips in circular movements avoiding the mouth, nostrils and eyes, working upwards and outwards. Remove with damp cotton wool and repeat.

- **Toning** is designed to remove any remaining cleanser and surface debris from the skin and helps to close the pores and refresh the skin. Using two pieces of damp cotton wool, apply a small amount of toner to the centre of the cotton wool and wipe gently over the neck and face. Allow to evaporate naturally from the skin or blot with tissue.

- **Moisturising** is the skin's food. It nourishes and helps to replace moisture that is lost from the skin during the cleansing procedure and the course of the day. Apply a small amount of moisturiser to the back of your non-working hand and transfer it to your palms. Using effleurage, apply to the neck and the face and gently massage in using your finger tips, making circular movements and working upwards and outwards.

Skin tones

There are at least 36 different African-Caribbean skin tones. The term 'African-Caribbean' is therefore used generally but the graduations of colour range from light brown/tan, mahogany/brown to ebony/black.

To enable all the various skin tones to be accommodated when selecting cosmetics, a good eye for colour and clever mixing of foundations and powders is necessary as the colour required may not always be found in one palette.

In some cases there might be a vast difference in pigmentation on the lips, in comparison with the natural skin colour. The lips may be lighter, darker or uneven in some areas. It would be fair to say that a characteristic of African-Caribbean skin is lip colour imbalance and the subtle application of a lip base (lip foundation) and lip colour can help to diminish this.

Differences between African-Caribbean and Caucasian skin

There are many differences between African-Caribbean and Caucasian skins, but the main and obvious difference is colour. All skins contain colour or pigment but it is the concentration of pigment in African-Caribbean skins that differs. African-Caribbean skins have some of their pigment at the skin's surface and that is why it is visible, making the skin darker. Caucasian skins have their pigment much deeper into the layers of the skin. Both African-Caribbean and Caucasian skins have pigment in the germinative layer of the epidermis but African-Caribbean skins have a greater concentration of pigment as opposed to Caucasian skins.

The table outlines the main differences between African-Caribbean and Caucasian skins. (See Chapter 2 for information on the structure of the skin.)

Typical skin disorders associated with African-Caribbean skins

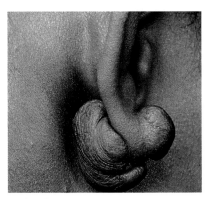

Keloid

Keloids

Keloids are overdeveloped, elevated scars. At first they may itch and feel tender, having a rubbery texture; later they become dense and hard. Keloids tend to occur as a result of the following types of skin injury:

- a burn or scald
- cuts or surgical wounds (e.g. an injection or skin incision)
- shaving or irritated ear piercing.

African-Caribbean skins	*Caucasian skins*
Desquamating cells contain pigmentary cells called melanocytes	Desquamating cells contain no melanocytes
Cells desquamate more frequently	Cells desquamate more slowly
Age at a slower rate	Age more rapidly
Have a thick horny layer	Have a thinner horny layer
Tan easily	Burn easily and tan more slowly because pigments are not superficial enough to provide protection
Produce large melanosomes	Produce very small melanosomes
Have larger and more numerous sebaceous glands per square centimetre on the face than Caucasian skins	Have 400–900 sebaceous glands per square centimetre on the face
Have one tenth of their sebaceous glands opening directly onto the skin's surface	
Have larger and more numerous sudoriferous glands per square centimetre on the face	Have 400–900 sudoriferous glands per square centimetre on the face
May have a lip colour imbalance	Even lip colour
Melanin naturally protects the skin and filters the sun's ultraviolet rays, capturing free radicals	Free radicals damage unprotected skin. The production of collagen and elastin is interrupted which leads to the deterioration of the skin, premature wrinkling and ageing

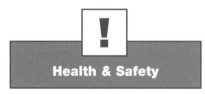

Health & Safety

These treatment methods are designed to reduce the size of the scarring but if applied incorrectly could also damage the skin surrounding the scar, causing the skin to become depressed therefore 're-elevating' the scar.

It is not possible to identify what type of scar will develop following injury and therefore keloids cannot be prevented. This type of scar can be removed surgically but the results are not always successful. Keloids tend to recur with a much more severe and unsightly appearance so alternative medical treatments are usually considered.

Treatments

- irradiation – applied under medical supervision in a hospital using X-rays, radioisotopes or other forms of ionising radiation
- local injections of cortisone – applied under medical supervision in a hospital

- local applications of cortisone tape – prescribed medical tape applied by the patient. (Cortisone is a steroid application that helps to reduce inflammation.)

Hyper-pigmentation

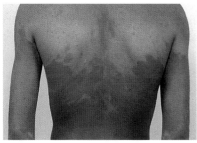

Hyper-pigmentation

When a skin injury such as a cut, spot or graze occurs, blood rushes to the injury site to help soothe and aid regeneration. In African-Caribbean traumatised skin, melanocytes also go to the injury site and therefore leave the affected area darker: this is known as **post-inflammatory hyper-pigmentation**. Once the healing process is completed, the excessive pigmentation will gradually fade, but not always back to the original skin colour.

Hyper-pigmentation may also occur when there is a build-up of dead skin cells, when the skin is dehydrated, following friction, e.g. scratching, and after some skin disorders, e.g. eczema, acne.

Hypo-pigmentation

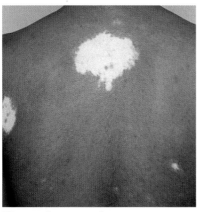

Hypo-pigmentation

Hypo-pigmentation is also known as **post inflammatory hypo-pigmentation**. This term refers to the loss of pigment at the site of an injury. In some cases the pigment loss can be permanent.

Complete pigment loss (when the melanocytes no longer produce melanin granules) is known as **vitiligo**. Vitiligo is not a systematic disease but a cosmetic disfigurement. The germinative layer of the epidermis no longer produces melanin, therefore leaving the skin sensitive to ultraviolet rays.

Hyper-keratinisation

Tip

Regular facials help in the removal of dead skin cells, and a lower build-up of dead skin cells results.

African-Caribbean skin cells are replaced much more rapidly than Caucasian skin cells but the dead cells are not always removed from the skin's surface at the same rate. This leads to a build-up of dead skin cells known as hyper-keratinisation, which in turn leads to hyper-pigmentation. To help alleviate these conditions on African-Caribbean skins thorough skincare is advised which should include cleansing, facial scrubs, face masks, toning and moisturising as part of a home-care and salon routine. This will aid the 'turnover' of the skin, removing the 'old' skin and allowing the 'new' skin to come to the surface.

The importance of analysing the skin

Tip

The thickness of African-Caribbean skin can vary from medium to thick due to the horny layer being considerably thicker.

Tip

African-Caribbean skin tends to have a greater secretion of oil than Caucasian skin due to its larger and more numerous sebaceous glands.

Prior to conducting any treatment, it is essential that a full assessment of the client's skin and related personal history is undertaken. This will enable the therapist to provide the best treatment for the client, ensuring that everything used is compatible with their needs and unlikely to cause irritation or side effects. It is not unusual for details of a confidential nature to be discussed and recorded. This information is for reference purposes only and should not be disclosed, i.e. treated as confidential.

At the start of a skin analysis, general information is required, i.e. full name, contact address and phone number(s). It is then necessary to establish details that cover the client's medical history as some conditions may contra indicate proposed treatments or may require clearance from the GP.

Certain personal habits may have a negative or positive effect on the condition of the skin and it is important that these are identified. For example, smoking, caffeine and alcohol are known to dehydrate the skin whereas exercise and fresh air stimulate the circulation, aiding regeneration. In some cases hormonal contraceptives and HRT can dry the skin and also stimulate abnormal hair growth as well as causing weight gain for some individuals.

Some questions may not appear relevant to the initial visit but they can be kept on file and referred to in future visits. Delicate questions, such as those that refer to HIV and Hepatitis B, are necessary as the knowledge of these conditions will ensure that a totally safe treatment is conducted, protecting the client, other clients, visitors and staff. The chart on the next page outlines the questions you should ask the client prior to undertaking any treatment.

Skin-care products should be selected to achieve the best results for each individual skin type. It is recommended to use products from one range as they will be compatible and designed to work together. The casual mixing of product ranges can lead to allergic reactions and poor performance.

African-Caribbean skin care and cosmetics

Prior to the application of make-up, it is necessary to carry out the usual cleansing procedure to provide a clean canvas to work on. Many products that are designed for African-Caribbean skins are called 'astringent' or 'oil-free'. Research

SKIN ANALYSIS/DIAGNOSIS PROCEDURE

Name: Contact No: Day:

                                                              Evening:

Home address:

Doctor's name: Contact No:

Address:

Medical history (operations in the last 12 months):
Medication taken within the last 6 months
(sedatives, anti-depressants, diuretics, laxatives):

Method of contraception:
Last pregnancy:
Hysterectomy: yes/no   if yes   Date:
HRT method:

Have you been tested for HIV/AIDS virus?   yes/no

Skin conditions/allergies
(eczema, psoriasis, acne):
Pore size (small, medium, large):
Skin texture (tight, smooth, uneven, coarse):
Skin thickness (fine, medium, thick):
Oil secretion:
Facial hair: yes/no   if yes   fine/downy/coarse?
Wrinkles: yes/no   if yes   where?
Pigmented areas:
Present skin condition:

Skin type: dry/normal/oily/combination/sensitive
                                               (may be a singular or combined skin type, e.g.
                                               dry/sensitive)

Do you smoke?   yes/no
Average per day:

Do you drink alcohol?   yes/no
Average weekly consumption:

Do you drink beverages containing caffeine?   yes/no
Average daily consumption:

Are you on a weight-reducing diet?   yes/no
Have you experienced any allergies to food?   yes/no

Do you take part in any aerobic or other
sporting activities?   yes/no

Client signature:

Therapist's name: signature:

has found that harsh astringents with no added oil can lead to dehydration and in African-Caribbean skins we know this can then lead to hyper-pigmentation. It would then appear quite important that some oil is used in these products and milder astringents should be considered to prevent dehydration of the skin.

As oils should be used in skin preparations it would be advisable to use an oil closer in composition to the skins natural oil, sebum. Mineral oils are usually the types used in skin-care preparations. Lanolin is added to mineral oils; it is a very good emollient but it is much denser than sebum and is also known to be the cause of some skin allergies. Protein oils are closer in density to sebum and this type of oil is less likely to clog the pores and cause comedones (blackheads).

Familiar African-Caribbean cosmetic companies

- E'ON 5 – African-Caribbean skin-care range
- Flori Roberts – cosmetics, camouflage make-up, skin-care products
- Sleek – cosmetics
- Fashion Flair – cosmetics and skin-care products
- Naomi Sims – cosmetics and skin-care products
- Paradise – cosmetics and skin care
- Black Radiance – cosmetics
- Iman – cosmetics.

Cosmetics for African-Caribbean skins have always been available but not always easily accessible. Only a matter of a few years ago, if you did not live in an area with a large African-Caribbean community you would have found it very difficult to purchase affordable, suitable products. Nowadays these products can be bought in familiar, local chemists and stores and the choices have greatly improved, with other well-known cosmetic houses now manufacturing make-up with suitable colours and foundations for African-Caribbean skins.

Differences between cosmetics for African-Caribbean and Caucasian skins

The main difference between the cosmetics is one of the main ingredients used to aid good coverage – **titanium**

dioxide. Though used widely in Caucasian powders and foundations, when used in African-Caribbean skin preparations the product's composition is too light and when applied to the skin it gives a sallow, ashy appearance. Make-up application methods will need to be adapted for your African-Caribbean clients and close attention must also be given to the colours chosen.

Facial characteristics of African-Caribbean and Caucasian clients differ in that your African-Caribbean clients will tend to have broader noses and fuller lips. Some African-Caribbean races have quite high cheek bones. If face shaping is required by your client you could consider:

- shading the sides of the nose to slim down its width and highlighting the tip
- using a lip defining pencil and lining slightly inside the natural lip line to reduce its fullness; using darker, matt lip shades
- shading the cheek bones to reduce their height and using darker, matt shades, avoiding glossy and glittery make-up which will emphasise the oil content of the skin (this will also apply to eye make-up).

Basically there are seven face shapes: oval, square, heart, round, long, pear and diamond (see also Chapter 6). The oval shape is recognised as the 'ideal' face shape. The other shapes are 're-shaped' using highlighting and shading to give them the appearance of the oval face. Other factors to take into consideration before carrying out face shaping are:

- eye colour
- hair colour
- hair style.

When deciding what face shaping is required, it is necessary to study the shape from the frontal and profile views and note the categories that most fit in with your client. These categories are:

- forehead – low or high
- eyes – close or wide set
- chin – receding or protruding
- nose – long or short, broad or slim
- lips – thin or full.

Highlighting is used to show up or emphasise features and **shading** is used to 'hide' or minimise features that are

Tip

It should be noted that most clients will be happy with their natural features and may not require shading.

less flattering. These effects can be achieved by using foundations, cover sticks, blushers and powders. The ideal choice of foundation for highlighting or shading should be either two or three shades lighter or darker than the 'correct' base shade. To achieve the best results from highlighting and shading, face shaping should be carried out after the application of the 'correct' foundation. If this method is carried out successfully there should be no obvious colour change; it should appear natural due to good blending.

The diagrams show the seven face shapes with the degree of highlighting and shading that is required to 'achieve' an oval face shape.

As previously identified, African-Caribbean clients will tend to have broader noses and fuller lips than Caucasian clients. The diagrams illustrate how to reduce the fullness of these features if required.

Highlighting and shading

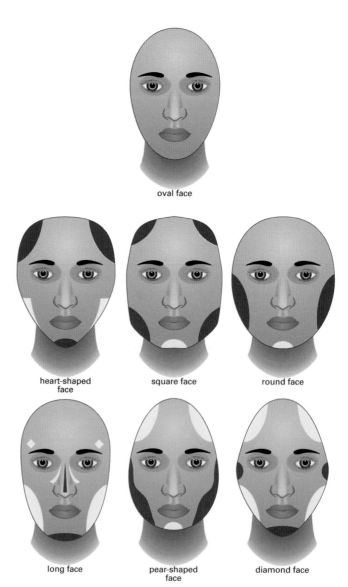

oval face

heart-shaped face

square face

round face

long face

pear-shaped face

diamond face

Eyebrows also play a part in the shape of the face and the emphasis of the eyes. Tweezing (in the direction of growth) can be used to re-shape the eyebrows; eyebrow tint may also be applied prior to tweezing. The application of eyebrow pencil can be used to emphasise the brows. Finally, brush the brows in the direction of their growth.

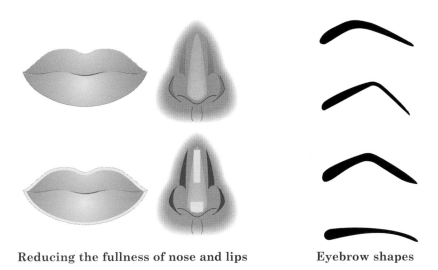

Reducing the fullness of nose and lips   Eyebrow shapes

Selecting the right colours for African-Caribbean skins

Avoid:

Pale, pastel shades, e.g. light pink, lime greens, pearlised, glitter shades during the day as they attract light emphasising the shine on some African-Caribbean skins

White, silver shades as they can be uncomplimentary on African-Caribbean clients unless applied skilfully and used as highlighters, to emphasise features

Lip gloss, as it emphasises the fullness of the lips

Choose from:

Dark, rich, vibrant colours
Earthy colours
Rusty, coppery colours
Deep berries
Browns, mahogany
Reds and burgundies
Purples, wines, deep coral
Orange, pinky reds
Matt colours, especially for the day as they do not reflect the light
Pearlised, glitter shades limited to evening make-up

African-Caribbean cosmetics:

Contain little or no titanium dioxide or zinc oxide (because they give an ashy appearance to African-Caribbean skin)
Favour fine, loose powders for adherence and absorbency
Have dark, rich, vibrant colours
Favour matt colours

Caucasian cosmetics:

Contain titanium dioxide or zinc oxide (because they aid good coverage)

Have pastel and some darker shades
May be matt, gloss or glitter

Basic make-up techniques

Tip

To achieve the best make-up results, the light should fall evenly onto the face.

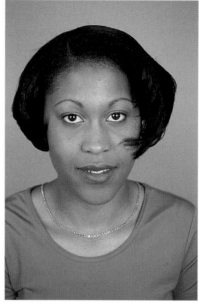

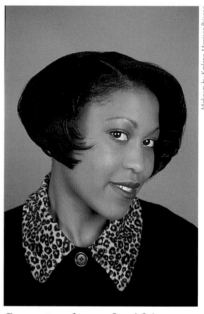

Make-up by Karlene Morrison-Briscoe

Caucasian make-up on African-Caribbean skin

Correct make-up for African-Caribbean skin

!

Health & Safety

Always wash hands thoroughly with an anti-bacterial liquid soap before touching the skin.

Tip

Make-up should be applied under the appropriate lighting conditions, e.g. daylight for daytime make-up and fluorescent light for evening make-up.

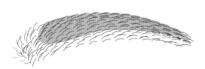

Eyebrow shaping

Before any make-up is applied, the skin needs to be prepared and all other traces of make-up removed. Cleanse, tone and moisturise the skin with the appropriate products for the skin type. Allow the moisturiser time to be absorbed into the skin before applying any make-up.

The selection of colours should be done now that the skin is clean and its true skin colour can be seen. If concealing work is required, the different colours of foundations can be chosen along with the foundation required for the whole face. To obtain the best colour match, the foundation should be tested along the jaw-line of the client; this gives the best match between the face and the neck. Work in good, even light, daylight is ideal for daytime make-up.

1   Shape the eyebrows if required. Tweeze the hairs in the direction of their growth, only removing hairs below the natural brow-line or between both eyebrows. When finished, wipe over with witch hazel to help soothe.

2   Carry out corrective make-up using concealer and/or foundation.

3   Apply the foundation to the whole face. Using a damp make-up wedge or natural sponge, dot the foundation onto the forehead, cheeks, nose and chin and begin to blend in an outward and downward direction, following

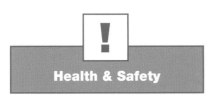

Health & Safety

All brushes, sponges and tools should be sanitised using brush cleanser or a similar preparation before they are re-used; where possible use disposable items.

the growth of the facial hairs to prevent them standing up and getting clogged. Keep the foundation thin and even. There is a choice between liquid, cream and mousse foundations or tinted moisturisers. The choice of foundation that you make will depend on your client. Is the client's skin greasy? If yes, try a liquid foundation as the oil content will be less than in a cream foundation. Are there very visible imperfections? Are you looking for good coverage? If yes, a cream foundation will give a more opaque coverage. Do you want a very thin coverage? If yes, choose from a liquid foundation or mousse, or even a tinted moisturiser as this will just give a lift to the client's own skin colour.

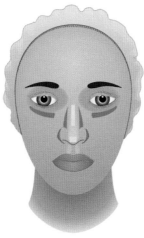

Applying corrective make-up

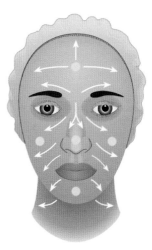

Applying and blending foundation

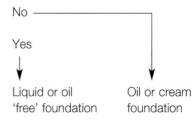

Is the client's skin greasy?

No ——————————
Yes
↓
Liquid or oil   Oil or cream
'free' foundation   foundation

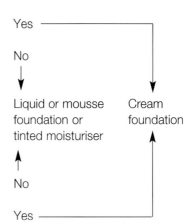

Are there visible imperfections?

Yes ——————————
No
↓
Liquid or mousse   Cream
foundation or   foundation
tinted moisturiser
↑   ↑
No
Do you want good coverage?
Yes ——————————

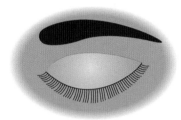

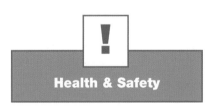

4   Powder is used to set the foundation. Remove some powder from the container using a clean spatula and transfer it to a clean make-up palette. Using three dry cotton wool disks or one new powder puff, work the powder into the powder puff and then gently rock the powdered puff over the face, pressing lightly to absorb the natural oils from the skin and set the foundation. As a result the foundation should appear matt and feel dry and smooth but not tacky. Now using one dry cotton wool disk, very gently repeat this technique over the eyelids and under the eye. Avoid applying excess powder to the eye area as this may emphasise fine lines and wrinkles. Finally, gently apply the puff across the lips; this will help to maintain the longevity of the lipstick. If required, use a clean powder brush to dust off any excess powder. This technique of powdering is very effective in maintaining a matt, shine-free foundation for a longer length of time and is also advisable for use on skins that have a tendency to be oily. There is a choice between translucent or opaque powders and loose or block powders. A translucent powder allows the colour of the foundation to show through. Opaque powders help with coverage and stop light getting through, therefore masking any imperfections. Loose powders tend to give a thinner coverage and are usually quite absorbent but a less experienced client might find them more difficult to handle at home and perhaps apply too much. In that case a block powder might be a good alternative as you only remove the amount you need.

5   **The eyes.**
Powdered shadows are best used on African-Caribbean skins that have a tendency to be more oily as they do not add to the oil already in the skin. To flatter the eyes, apply the darker shade to the inner and outer corners of the lids with a small amount of highlighter across the centre of the lid and into the arch of the eyebrow. Blend well. If you choose to use cream shadows or blusher they should be applied first and the powdered shadow/blusher applied on top to set. This gives a stronger and longer lasting colour.
Eyeliner For a softer look apply some eye shadow (black or dark grey) along the line of the eye and gently smudge. Alternatively, use a soft eyeliner pencil or eye liner block – damp an eye liner brush and smudge to achieve a similar effect. For a more defined look, use a pointed eyeliner pencil or liquid liner.
Eyebrows If definition is required or perhaps the eyebrows need lengthening, use an eyebrow brush and an eyebrow pencil to match the client's eyebrows. Brush

some colour on to the bristles of the brush. Now brush the colour through the brows and extend their length if needed. Use the pencil to do the finishing touches to the shape. Blend again with the brush if needed. By using a brush rather than the pencil on its own the application is less heavy, giving a more natural look.

6 Blusher should be applied from the top of the cheek bone, near the ear, down to the base of the bone, level with the tip of the nose. For emphasis, apply blusher on the bone and use a darker colour underneath the bone.

7 To counteract any lip colour imbalance and also to help give longevity to lipstick, foundation can be applied to the lips at the foundation stage or a lip base (a foundation for the lips) can be applied now. If the lips are full, apply the lip liner (choose a colour similar to the lipstick) slightly inside the natural line of the lips (see page 289). To give a richer colour to the lipstick and also to help with its staying power, lip pencil can be applied to the whole lip. Using a lip brush, apply the chosen lipstick, keeping inside the new lip line.

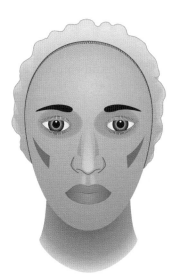

Applying blusher

The following photographs show three different looks that can be achieved with make-up.

Natural look
Foundation: light base
Blusher: natural beech
Eyeshadow: light brown
Eyeliner: brown
Mascara: black – light application

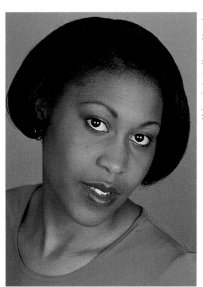

Makeup by Jessica Yongze Nyoledzy

Natural look

Fashion look
Foundation: heavier base
Blusher: plum
Eyeshadow: gold/yellow on the lids brought out at the sides of the eye; brown on the sockets
Eyeliner: black
Mascara: black built up to three coats
Lipstick: plum glossy

Glamour look
Foundation: heavier base
Blusher: plum
Eyeshadow: silvery deep blue in sockets and lids; glitter on brow-line
Eyeliner: black solid line
Mascara: black applied heavily
Lipstick: deep purple lipstick and lipliner

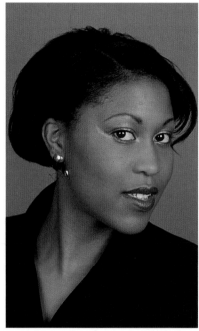 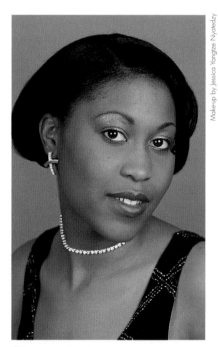

Make-up by Jessica Yangtze Nyatedzy

Fashion look   Glamour look

Glossary of skin and make-up terms

Astringent a strong toning lotion with a high proportion of alcohol

Comodones (blackheads) dried sebum or keratin scales in the mouth of the hair follicle. Oxidisation by the oxygen in the air turns the plug 'black'

Cortisone steroid based product

Dehydration loss of water/moisture from the skin

Desquamation (shedding) skin cells coming off in scales

Emollient minute droplets of one insoluble liquid suspended in another insoluble liquid

Free radicals highly reactive molecules which cause skin cells to degenerate

Hyper-keratosis overgrowth of the horny layer

Hyper-keratinisation a build up of dead skin cells

Hyper-pigmentation the accumulation of pigment in a area resulting in localised darkening of skin

Hypo-pigmentation localised pigment loss at the site of an injury

Keloids overdeveloped, raised, dense scar; may feel tender and itchy

Malignant melanoma a type of skin cancer often recognised by a change in the normal appearance and/or feel of the skin or mole – a change in the size, colour or texture of the mole

Melanocytes granules of yellow, brown or black pigment (melanin) produced by melanocytes

Sebaceous glands oil glands

Sudoriferous glands sweat glands

Titanium dioxide added to make-up preparations to produce a more opaque product and also to increase the covering power

Traction alopecia hair loss caused by harsh treatment of the hair, for example by brushing vigorously

Health and safety

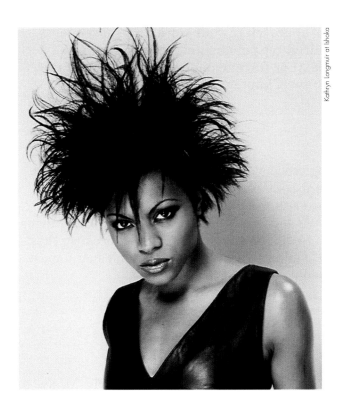

15

Kathryn Longmuir at Ishoka

Learning objectives

This chapter covers the following:

- **personal hygiene**
- **hygiene in the salon**
- **health and safety legislation**
- **non-infectious disorders**
- **infectious factors**
- **hair loss**
- **animal parasites**

Personal hygiene

Image is of great importance within the hairdressing industry. First impressions always count and clients usually make a visual judgement on your ability and the type of service they are about to receive. At all times you should aim to be professional and maintain a high standard, as this reflects your approach to your work and subsequently attracts the required type of clientele. It also shows self-respect and pride. (For further information on appearance and presentation see Chapter 1.)

Body Care

Regular cleansing twice a day together with anti-perspirant deodorants prevent body odour and control perspiration. Showers are quicker than baths and more hygienic. Whilst washing you should concentrate on genital areas, under arms and the feet. The feet have a tendency to smell because they have more sweat glands and breed bacteria, and spend most of the day enclosed in shoes.

Skin

Some general tips on skin maintenance:

- Cleanse, tone and moisturise skin regularly. Many moisturisers now offer protection against harmful UVA and UVB rays.
- Regular facials remove dead skin and control spots.
- Optionally you can tidy eyebrows, facial hair and wear light make-up.

(For further information on skin care and make-up see Chapter 14.)

Hair care

Hair should be clean, trimmed, healthy and always neat. The style should be modern and current. Clients depend on their stylists to keep them up to date with the new trends. Unkempt hair could reflect a negative attitude.

- As a *Health and Safety Regulation*, long hair should be tied back to avoid becoming tangled in equipment and falling over clients.
- Hair should be washed regularly to prevent it becoming lank and to reduce sebum on the forehead.

Oral care

Halitosis or unpleasant breath is more often than not a direct result of bad oral hygiene and can be caused by the following:

- not cleaning the teeth and mouth sufficiently, leaving food trapped between teeth
- eating strong-smelling or highly seasoned foods, such as garlic, onions, coffee
- not visiting the dentist regularly to identify dental problems
- smoking
- digestive problems
- not eating regularly.

Hands

You create with your hands, so they must be well cared for at all times. Cuts should be kept covered until healed. Warts should be medically removed. Nails should be regularly manicured to prevent nail breakage. Chipped nails may scratch your clients and tear and pull their hair. Chipped nail varnish looks untidy and unprofessional – it is easy and quick to remove it.

Continuous use of shampoos and hair-processing chemicals can cause **contact dermatitis** – the skin becomes inflamed with a dry, irritable rash that spreads rapidly, in extreme cases covering the entire body. This can permanently damage and discolour the skin and nails. It is a *Health and Safety Regulation* and also very sensible if you wish to engage in a long career in hairdressing, to protect and cover hands with continuous use of barrier creams and protective gloves.

Clothes

As with the hair, clean, neat, comfortable and fashionable clothes help to complete the picture of a positive attitude and a person who pays attention to fashion. Natural fibres such as cotton and linen are preferable as they allow the skin to breathe and will not absorb body odour. Clothes should not be revealing and underarms should be covered. In some establishments it may be a requirement to wear a uniform, to promote a corporate image. The uniform should be worn with pride and not grudgingly.

Jewellery

Jewellery (such as rings and chains) should be kept to a minimum as it could catch on clients' hair when carrying out salon services. It could also tarnish whilst using chemicals.

Footwear

Footwear for the salon must be comfortable and easy to clean, low heeled and made of natural fibres such as leather, to allow the feet to breathe. Fashionable shoes are not always designed for comfort and can cause the feet to become increasingly painful after hours of standing.

High heels throw the body forward and can lead to bad posture and fatigue of the feet. Low or medium heels are more comfortable, the shoe should grip the heel and cover the instep and toes to prevent entry of stray hairs into the skin. Sensible footwear and possibly support tights, can help prevent the feet aching and ankles swelling after a long day spent standing.

Feet should be washed regularly.

Posture

Standing for long periods of time causes tired feet, swollen ankles and backache amongst other things. Hairdressers tend to suffer from either one or all of these ailments. The way a person stands, sits and walks is known as posture. A hairdresser must take note of his/her posture in order to reduce aches and permanent injury. An individual's posture depends on the skeleton, ligaments which hold it together and the muscles which help movement. Good posture means that the muscles do not tire easily and cause damage and injury.

Whilst standing you should:

- stretch the body upwards
- position the spine in a natural curl
- contract the stomach muscles to keep the back erect
- distribute the body-weight onto both feet, shoulder width apart
- wear low-heeled shoes to reduce pressure on legs and ankles.

Hairdressing is a standing job, and does tend to cause swelling of feet and eventually varicose veins in the legs.

This is because in walking, the action of the leg muscles helps to return circulation of blood and lymph from the feet and legs. By just standing this action is not occurring, so blood and lymph tend to accumulate in the feet and lower legs, causing swelling.

Exercise in one way of controlling the swelling. Brisk walking and cycling not only strengthen muscles, but also aid in improving circulation. Whenever possible, always try to elevate feet as this helps the blood flow.

Hygiene in the salon

The salon environment, including backstage, should be kept as clean as possible at all times. The following guides are procedures that should be carried out daily or whenever something needs cleaning.

All **floors** should be:

- made of a non-slip surface, i.e. vinyl, which is easily cleaned
- clean at all times – regularly mopped, swept and/or vacuumed
- marked by a visible notice when cleaning is in progress
- cleared of hair – hair should be swept regularly and placed in covered bins.

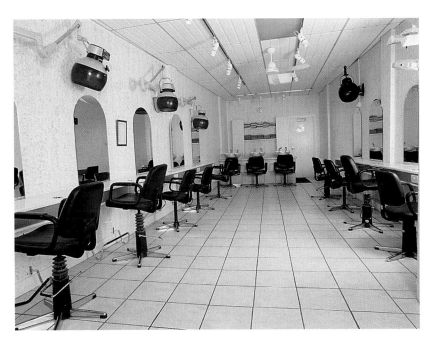

A modern salon

Chairs should be:

- made of a washable fabric, i.e. vinyl, or any fabric that is easily wiped
- washed with a detergent daily
- wiped with alcohol or disinfectant daily.

Trolleys should:

- be clean
- have removable trays – preferably plastic
- be washed with detergent daily.

Rollers and **perm rods** should:

- be cleaned after each use, i.e. hair removed and disinfected or washed in detergent
- be sorted into colours, sizes and shapes or types, etc.

Mirrors should be:

- cleaned daily with glass cleaner and/or hot water.

All **reading material** (literature and magazines) should be:

- current and appropriate to suit clientele
- kept tidy in a rack and free from damage if possible.

Hairdressing tools and equipment

- **Gowns** must be washed daily.
- **Towels** must be washed after every use in hot soapy water to remove soils and smells and to kill germs and thereby prevent the spread of infection.

Tools

Ideally, tools should be used on just one client, then cleansed and sterilised before use with the next client. Tools that fall on the floor must be cleaned and sterilised before they are used again and placed in the tool bag to avoid contamination.

Metal surgical instruments, i.e. scissors and razors, are cleaned by wiping with an antiseptic swab or surgical spirit.

Tip

When sterilising combs and brushes use the following procedure:
- remove all hair
- wash in warm, soapy water
- soak in disinfectant
- rinse before use.
Always follow manufacturer's instructions on the use of disinfectants.

Sterilisation

Sterilisation is the complete destruction of all living organisms on an object. However, once sterilised items are exposed to the air they are no longer sterile. The process can be carried out in four ways: heat, vapour, chemicals and radiation.

Heat

Heat sterilisation can either be by dry or moist heat.

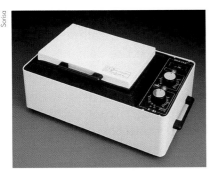

A dry heat sterilising cabinet

- **Dry:** One method is the use of a dry, hot air oven. The heat reaches a temperature between 150 and 180°C, and has to be maintained for 30–60 minutes without disturbance. This method is not normally used today. A modern method is a **glass bead steriliser**. This type is excellent for small tools, which are placed on electrically heated small beads. These channel heat to objects placed on them.

- **Moist:** Moist heat sterilisation is the process of steaming tools under pressure (autoclave) using the same principles as a pressure cooker (see diagram). The units are automatic and increase the pressure on water to 32 lb/in² which raises the boiling temperature to 134°C. This means complete sterilisation only takes 3–4 minutes; tools can be returned for use very quickly. Although this method is very effective it could cause rusting and distort plastics.

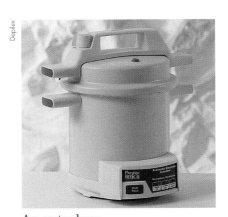

An autoclave

Vapour

The gases used in vapour cabinets include ethylene oxide and formaldehyde. These are too hazardous to use, so therefore other methods have now replaced this method.

Chemicals

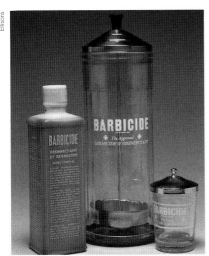

Barbicide

- **Disinfectants:** These liquids destroy a large majority of micro-organisms. Solutions such as quarternary ammonium compounds (quats) or glutaraldehyde (e.g. Barbicide). work against bacteria and fungi to remove contamination by coating them or drying them out. They are very suitable for salon use and chemicals can be added which inhibit rust, thus making disinfectants suitable for most tools.

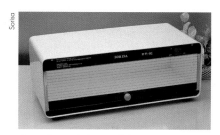

An ultraviolet cabinet

- **Antiseptics:** These liquids prevent the rapid growth of micro-organisms but are not permanent and do not kill micro-organisms. They are kinder than disinfectants and effective enough to be used on the skin.

Radiation

Ultraviolet rays destroy micro-organisms. They are produced artificially by mercury vapour lamps. The UV rays are harmful to skin and eyes. In modern cabinets, the UV lamp automatically switches off when the door is opened.

Germs absorb the radiation and die, but as ultraviolet light travels in straight lines, the tools must be turned after 20 minutes, even then the rays do not get into the corners. Although anything can be sterilised by ultraviolet, it is time-consuming and not very effective. Before sterilisation, tools must be washed to remove grease which will protect germs.

Ventilation

Ventilation is the process by which stale air is replaced by fresh air. Humans alter the composition of the air in the salon by breathing and perspiration. The oxygen in the air will be reduced whilst the carbon dioxide will increase. This leads to feelings of exhaustion and sluggishness. Ventilation in the salon, either naturally or mechanically, helps reduce the high levels of humidity which can prevent the body from cooling itself properly.

Natural ventilation

Natural ventilation is when gases in the air move naturally, i.e. by draughts. The air should be changed three or four times an hour. The cool air must not enter the room below shoulder level and should be directed upwards.

Two similar methods of ventilation without draughts are:

- a **coopers' disc** provides some control of the incoming air. The inner disc is rotated so that its holes coincide with similar holes in the window.
- **louvred windows** consist of movable strips of glass which may be used as air inlets or outlets according to their position.

Artificial ventilation

Artificial ventilation is commonly known as air conditioning. The air moves freely by itself and does not need any special treatment. Efficiency is calculated by multiplying the room volume by the number of complete air changes required per hour.

Fans

- Room fans do not ventilate, they only circulate air.
- Extractor fans remove fumes and dust from the air, but do not ventilate.

Health and Safety legislation

The **Health and Safety at Work Act 1974** ensures that all business premises and equipment are safe and in excellent working order.

- The temperature in the salon should be maintained at a minimum of 16°C. With adequate ventilation, the levels of carbon dioxide can be controlled, reducing the effects of nausea. Limited ventilation causes many chemicals to become hazardous.
- The premises should be well lit, to ensure all treatments are executed with the minimum possibility of causing an accident.
- Toilets and hand-washing facilities must be provided.

Any accidents, major or minor, occurring in the salon to staff and clients must be recorded in an **accident book** (see example). The following information must be clearly recorded in the book:

- casualty's full name and address
- entry date
- date of the accident
- full details of the accident and location
- injury sustained
- details of action taken
- signature of person making entry.

In addition, it is also important to keep a record of any injuries, burns, etc. sustained during any services provided by the salon. This is of importance should the client pursue the matter.

Example of accident book layout

Date of entry	
Casualty name Address & telephone	
Accident full description	
Injury sustained & action taken	Name & signature of recorder

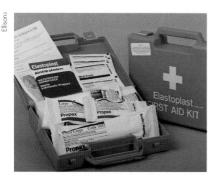

A first-aid box

First aid box

There should be a first-aid trained member of staff on the premises at all times during opening hours. Sufficient first aid boxes should be positioned in accessible locations, the contents of which should be according to current **Health and Safety (First Aid) Regulations 1981**:

- basic first-aid guidance leaflet (1)
- individually wrapped sterile adhesive dressings (20)
- individually wrapped triangular bandages (6)
- safety pins (6)
- sterile eye-pads, with attachments (2)
- medium-sized, individually wrapped, sterile, un-medicated wound dressing – 10 cm × 8 cm (6)
- large, individually wrapped, sterile, un-medicated wound dressings – 13 cm × 9 cm (2)
- extra-large, sterile, individually wrapped, medicated wound dressings – 28 cm × 17.5 cm (3)

Eyes can be rinsed out with tap water; alternatively, sterile water contained in sealed containers is just as good.

Electricity at Work Regulations 1989

This regulation states that all electrical equipment should be tested by a qualified electrician every 12 months. A visual inspection can be carried out on a regular basis by designing your own checklist. Be aware of potential hazards:

- frayed cables
- broken or cracked plugs

- overloaded sockets
- exposed wires in flexes.

Control of Substances Hazardous to Health (COSHH) Regulations 1999

These regulations help control employers' exposure to hazardous substances, whilst allowing them to assess any possible risk to health. Substances need to be stored in the correct manner, otherwise it can prove to be quite hazardous. All hazardous substances should be clearly labelled with symbols and it is important to store and handle them correctly.

A hazardous substance can get into the body via:

- the skin
- the eyes
- the nose (breathed in)
- the mouth (swallowed).

It is the hairdressing product supplier's responsibility to provide adequate information on how the materials should be used and stored. These forms are always available on request.

The Personal Protective Equipment at Work Regulations 1992 (PPE)

These regulations, guarded by COSHH, ensure employers provide adequate personal protective equipment (for example, the use of gloves when handling perm lotion) for handling hazardous substances in the salon such as:

- acid solutions in different strengths
- alkaline creams in different strengths
- vapour and colouring agents
- pressurised cans filled with flammable liquid.

Handling of tools needs extreme caution and adequate training. Examples are:

- heated appliances
- electrical appliances
- sharp cutting tools.

The employer also has the responsibility to ensure staff are trained correctly to use PPE (personal protective equipment).

The Health and Safety at Work Act is enforced by the Local Authority Environment Health Department, who authorises environmental health officers to inspect local business premises. If the inspector recognises a potential danger, the employer is issued with an improvement notice, which allows a designated time for improvements. If the improvements are not carried out accordingly, the inspector will then issue a prohibition notice, and could close the business until such dangers have been made safe for employees and the public.

The Fire Precaution Act 1971

This act states that all employees should receive adequate training in fire and emergency evacuation procedures. The emergency exit is the shortest and quickest exit for staff and clients to leave the premises. A smoke alarm should be fitted to alert staff to any fires. A fire door could be fitted, to help contain the spread of fires.

Fire-fighting equipment should be stored conveniently around the building. The equipment should include fire blankets, fire extinguishers, buckets and water hoses. Do NOT use fire extinguishers unless you have been fully trained. It is important to know which extinguisher to use on a fire – using the wrong one could make matters worse. Always try to find the source of the fire.

- Fire blankets smother small fires or a person's clothes.
- Sand absorbs spilt liquids – if it is the source of the fire, smother the flames.
- Water hoses extinguish large fires caused by paper.

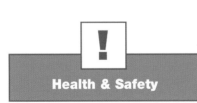

Health & Safety

In the event of a fire, if a chemical application has been started on a client and the salon has to be evacuated, find a salon or a neighbouring business where the products can be rinsed out safely.

Health & Safety

1997 European regulations have made all fire extinguishers red, with different coloured labels. Exercise extreme caution when selecting a fire extinguisher.

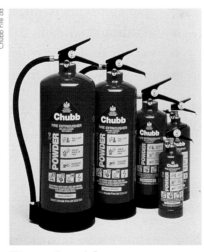

Fire extinguishers

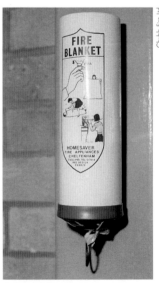

A fire blanket

Emergency numbers

It is good practice to have all emergency numbers listed and positioned in several easily accessible places, for example beside the till, on the staff room notice board, beside the telephone.

Non-infectious disorders

Several disorders of the hair and scalp are common and not contagious.

Disorders of the hair

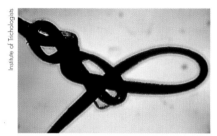

Monilethrix

Monilethrix

This is a fairly rare hereditary condition in which the thickness of the hair shaft varies along its length, caused by rapid changes in the hair growth cycle. The hair then takes on a beaded effect, making it weak and very brittle.

Trichonodosis

This term refers to knotting of the hair. Knotting occurs at the point where the hair shaft leaves the follicle. It can be seen as knots or loops in the hair and is caused by rough handling.

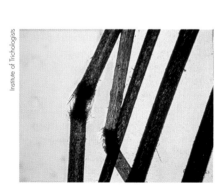

Trichorrhexis nodosa

Trichorrhexis nodosa

This condition is characterised by nodes or small split swellings on the hair shaft. The nodes resemble two brushes facing each other with their bristles interlocked. They are weak points along the shaft and the hair tends to break at these locations.

It is caused by rough handling or the use of strong hairdressing chemicals. The cuticle of the hair is damaged, moisture seeps into the cortex and damages the fibres, causing further splitting and damage. Gentler handling and treatment with oily conditioners should prevent further damage. This condition is more common in African-Caribbean hair than in Caucasian hair.

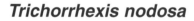

Fragilitas crinium

Fragilitas crinium

Known commonly as **split ends**. If the hair becomes dry and brittle it can split either at the ends or at various

Disorders of the hair

Disorder	Definition	Location	Cause	Sign	Treatment
Canities	Grey or white hair	Mainly seen on scalp and facial hair	Lack of pigment produced by the melanocytes in the hair follicle resulting in a mixture of coloured and white hair	White hair (may appear grey due to a mix of natural colour and white hair)	No treatment apart from permanent colouring
Monilethrix	Beaded hair	Occipital area	Uneven development of keratin	The hair shaft consists of irregular lumps resembling a row of beads	Massage and gentle handling of hair
Trichorrhexis nodosa	Nodules on hair shaft containing split hair	Middle lengths and ends	Physical or chemical damage	Nodules containing split and damaged hair swell lengthways along the hair shaft	Cut the damaged area off
Ringed hair	White coloured rings	Along the hair shaft	Uneven development of colour pigment in the production of keratin	Alternate rings of white and coloured hair	Deep reconstruction treatments
Damaged cuticle	Dry, broken hair	Middle lengths and ends of hair shaft	Physical or chemical damage to cuticle surface	The hair will have a dull appearance and the cuticle layer will be broken, torn and rough to touch	Cut damaged hair; apply semi-permanent to add sheen to dull hair
Fragilitas crinium	Split ends	Ends or points of hair	Physical and chemical damage, and rough handling of hair	Thin, split, weak frayed ends	Cut off damaged hair and apply deep conditioning treatment

points along the shaft. The condition is caused by either mechanical or chemical damage. Examples are perming, tinting or bleaching the hair too frequently, handling the hair too roughly (blow-drying, combing, etc.). Such treatment can damage the cuticle of the shaft, leading to splitting and fraying of the long, cylindrical, cortical fibres.

Split ends cannot be repaired. They may, however, be made to cling together by the use of some types of protein conditioners. This gives an electrostatic effect. The split ends should ideally be cut off. Beneficial treatments for people who suffer from split ends include hot oil treatments and cetrimide conditioners. The hair should be handled gently.

Disorders of the sebaceous gland

Seborrhoea

This term is used to describe an extremely greasy condition of the skin and scalp. It is caused by over-activity of the sebaceous glands and may be accompanied by pityriasis and areas of acne. Increased sebaceous gland activity commences at puberty and has been shown to be influenced by an increase in hormones. Hormone secretion usually becomes static by the age of 25. (For further information see Chapter 2.)

The hair becomes greasy and lank within a few days of washing. The scalp and face (particularly the forehead and nose) are also greasy. Vigorous brushing and massaging of the scalp increases the activity of the sebaceous glands and should be avoided or reduced to a minimum.

The condition can be controlled but not cured by using specially formulated shampoos. These shampoos are available from pharmacists and should be used twice a week. (See table for other disorders of the sebaceous glands.)

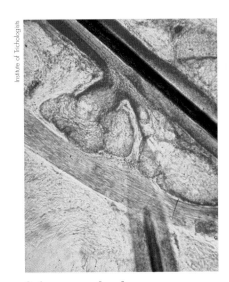

Sebaceous gland

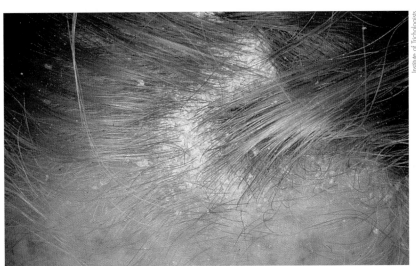

Seborrhoea dermatitis

Disorders of the scalp

Pityriasis

This is known as **dandruff** and is the most common scalp disorder. The dry, upper cells of the epidermis are constantly being shed, producing scales. The scales are shed

Disorders of the sebaceous glands

Disorder	Definition	Location	Cause	Signs	Treatment
Seborrhoea	Excessive greasiness of the skin and hair	Scalp, forehead and nose	Over-active sebaceous glands produce excessive amounts of sebum	Lank, limp, greasy hair, shiny, oily skin and moist to touch	Regulate and control oil production by keeping scalp, hair and skin clean; also by reducing physical or chemical stimulation; seek medical advice if symptoms continue
Acne	A disorder of the hair follicle and sebaceous glands	Face (forehead, cheeks) and upper back	Over-production of sebum which blocks the hair follicle opening; onset at puberty; related to hormone changes	Raised spots containing white pus and black-heads; the skin can become inflamed, irritated and sore; scarring and disfigurement are very common	Seek medical attention
Sebaceous cyst	Swelling of a sebaceous gland	Anywhere on the body	Sebum becomes trapped in the sebaceous duct, causing swelling anywhere from the size of a pea to a ping-pong ball	Bumps, lumps or swellings, soft to the touch, on the scalp which may be devoid of hair	Contents need to removed by a doctor
Seborrhoea dermatitis	A greasy form of dandruff	Around the hairline, seborrhoea areas (around the nose and behind the ears)	Excessive production of sebum accompanied by the over-production of epidermal cells; an allergic reaction to production of sebum	A yellow greyish greasy scale that covers the skin; the skin becomes red and extends beyond the scales; hairline often referred to as festoon (a chain of flowers)	Seek medical attention

from the scalp at an uncharacteristically high rate. It often starts in small itchy patches which spread to cover the whole scalp.

The condition may be temporary, permanent or intermittent. Although nothing can be done to actually cure it, the condition can be controlled by the use of anti-dandruff shampoos. These work by causing the upper layer of the epidermis to be shed during shampooing; the scales being washed out during rinsing. Depending on the severity of the dandruff, the scales should not show again for a few days.

Contact dermatitis may develop from prolonged use of anti-dandruff shampoos. It is always sensible to alternate between two different types of shampoo.

One of the most common active ingredients in anti-dandruff shampoos is a chemical called zinc pyrithione. The other chemical which will remove the keratin scales is selenium sulphide. This has the advantage of increasing sebaceous gland activity so is useful for very dry scalps. In extreme cases of scaling, keratolytic (keratin-splitting) ointments containing salicylic acid may be used.

Medicated shampoos do not stop scaling but are of use in keeping infections (caused by scratching) to a minimum. (For further information see Chapter 3.)

Psoriasis

This is a scaly condition of the skin. The keratin scales are dull and silvery, covering reddish lesions. Small bleeding points may occur if the scales are removed.

The disease is thought to occur in about 1 or 2% of the population and usually appears for the first time between the ages of 5 to 25. Girls suffering from psoriasis outnumber boys by 2 to 1, however by adult life, 40% of sufferers are men. The disease is less common in the summer.

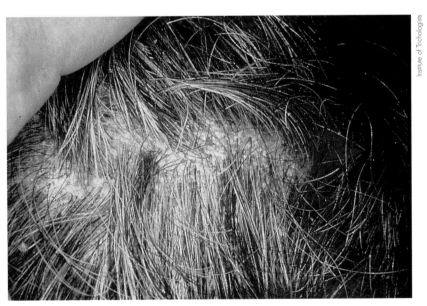

Psoriasis

Although the cause is unknown, there are several factors which influence its onset, the most important being heredity. The risk of psoriasis for children of one affected parent is about 25%. In about half of the cases of acute psoriasis during childhood, the onset of the disease can be linked to streptococcal tonsillitis. The psoriasis occurs within 10 to 14 days of the bacterial infection (suggesting an allergic response).

Mental stress is not a common factor in precipitating the first attack of psoriasis, but it is an undoubted influence on subsequent attacks.

On the scalp, the scales may be anchored by hair, allowing them to accumulate so that they can be easily located by touch. Although the condition may look unpleasant, normal hairdressing processes may be carried out once the psoriasis is no longer in an active state, i.e. no sore or broken skin on the scalp.

Disorders of the scalp

Disorder	Definition	Location	Cause	Signs	Treatment
Pityriasis capitis	Dandruff – dry scaling scalp	Scalp	Excessive production of epidermal cells which triggers the onset of bacterial or fungal infections	Dry flakes in patches accumulated around the scalp; eventually overall flaking; profound itching may be experienced	Regulate and control epidermal cell production by frequent shampooing with mild anti-dandruff shampoos; seek medical attention in severe cases
Psoriasis	An accumulation of scales on scalp/skin	Scalp, elbow and knees	Can be genetic, caused by an increase in cell production. Stress-related, non-infectious	Patches of silvery scales, thicker and larger than normal cells; once removed the skin appears red and may even bleed at these points	Seek medical attention
Eczema – dermatitis	At its simplest state, red inflamed skin	Anywhere on the body	Several external or internal factors; it may be a physical irritant or an allergic reaction	They range from a light redness to weeping, swelling, splitting of the skin and severe scaling, irritation and blisters; in chronic cases the underlying skin becomes infected	Seek medical attention

Infectious factors

The human body is host to a large number of micro-organisms. Some are harmless, non-pathogens and some are harmful pathogens, i.e. they are responsible for infections and disease. They are so small that only large colonies are visible to the naked eye under a powerful microscope.

Three types of pathogens are of great importance to the hairdresser:

- bacteria
- fungi
- viruses.

Bacteria

Bacteria are micro-organisms that inhabit the surface of the skin and hair. They reproduce rapidly when their surrounding conditions are favourable. They like the alkaline environment of body tissue and blood.

Bacteria multiply by cell division (mitosis). They need seven requirements to multiply:

- food
- moisture
- time
- warmth
- oxygen
- darkness
- alkalinity.

Bacteria can be either aerobic or anaerobic. Aerobic bacteria use atmospheric oxygen, whereas anaerobic bacteria can live without oxygen. Most bacteria thrive at a temperature of 37°C. Higher temperatures usually kill bacteria but they can form spores which can survive high temperatures. Bacterial spores are the last things to be destroyed during sterilisation.

Bacteria are classified according to shape:

- diplococci: round in pairs – pneumonia
- streptococci: round in chains – sore throats, impetigo
- staphylococci: round in bunches – boils, folliculitis
- bacilli: rod-shaped – typhoid fever (*Bacillus typhosus*), diphtheria

- spirochaetes: spiral-shaped – syphilis
- vibrios: comma-shaped – cholera

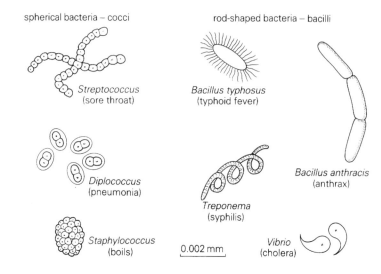

spherical bacteria – cocci

Streptococcus
(sore throat)

Diplococcus
(pneumonia)

Staphylococcus
(boils)

rod-shaped bacteria – bacilli

Bacillus typhosus
(typhoid fever)

Bacillus anthracis
(anthrax)

Treponema
(syphilis)

0.002 mm

Vibrio
(cholera)

Examples of bacteria

Name	Cause	Appearance	Site of infection	Treatment
Sycosis barbae, known as razor bumps, barber's rash or itch	Bacterial infection of hair follicles in the beard area	Small spots and blisters, inflamed, with burning sensations	Cheeks, and around the mouth	Medication must be prescribed; seek medical advice
Folliculitis	A bacterial infection of the hair follicles	Small spots around mouth of the hair follicle, raised and very sore	Hairy parts of the body, also seen around the nape area	As above
Furuncles (boils)	An infection of a follicle by staphylococci	Spots become raised, inflamed and painful, filled with pus	Commonly seen on the back of the neck	As above
Impetigo	A bacterial infection of the skin	Blisters appear around the mouth; eventually they burst to form a yellow crust	Most commonly seen around the mouth, nose and ears but can spread to the scalp or limbs	As above

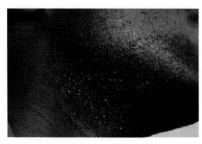

Sycosis barbae

Types of infectious bacteria

In-growing hairs

Removing curly or wavy hair against the natural growth pattern causes the hair to be pulled out of the hair follicle. The clubbed hair then springs back into its natural curl

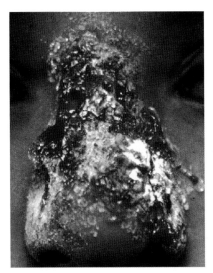

Impetigo

pattern and lies deeper in the hair follicle. The hair begins to grow into the follicle walls, and beneath the epidermis. The hair follicle becomes infected by staphylococcal bacteria. This infection causes raised, pus-filled spots and inflamed skin. This condition is highly contagious and can affect any hairy part of the body. It is common on the face in areas where hair grows, predominantly in African-Caribbean males.

Other common types of contagious bacterial infections related to hairdressing are outlined in the table on page 316.

Fungi

There are two types of pathogenic fungi which can live off the skin and give rise to disease:

- **Filamentous fungi** grow as fine, branching threads which invade and digest the keratin of skin, hair and nails. They tend to spread in a circular patch from where the original spore germinated, hence the common name **ringworm**.
- **Yeasts** are clusters of single-celled fungi which tend to invade the mucus membranous skin around the mouth or, in women, the vagina, to produce the disease, **thrush**.

Name	*Appearance*	*Site of infection*	*Treatment*
Tinea capitis, a fungal infection of the scalp; most common in children and can be caught directly from infected scalps	A bald patch on the scalp with some broken hairs, the scalp covered with greyish white scales; degree of disruption depends on the species of fungus	Scalp	Medical – griseofulvin
Tinea barbae, a fungal infection of the beard; can be spread by the use of infected tools	A group of small boils with broken hairs projecting from the heads	Beard area	Medical
Tinea pedis or **athlete's foot**, a fungal infection of the foot	Small blisters which burst, causing the skin to become scaly	In between the webs of the fourth and fifth toe	Medical – special foot powders and creams are available from the chemist
Tinea ungium, a fungal infection of the fingernails	The plate looks yellowish-grey. the weakened nail is brittle and lifts away from the nail plate	The nail plate	Medical – application of fungicides

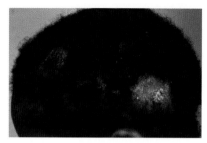

Tinea

Ringworm can affect different areas of the body; these conditions are not in themselves different but simply different medical descriptions of the areas affected:

- capitis – ringworm of the scalp
- barbae – ringworm of the beard
- pedis – ringworm of the feet
- ungium – ringworm of the toe- or fingernails.

These infections are described in the table on page 317.

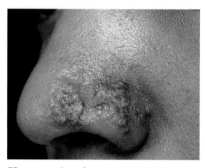

Herpes simplex

Viruses

Virus are minute organisms that invade and multiply inside a healthy body cell. The cell wall eventually ruptures and viral particles invade neighbouring cells, spreading the infection. Three common, contagious viral infections are described in the table opposite.

Acquired immune deficiency syndrome (AIDS)

Aids is the newest and most deadly virus condition known to man. It was first reported in 1981 and was given the name 'acquired immune deficiency syndrome'. The virus responsible is the human immunodeficiency virus (HIV).

The virus has been found in human blood, semen and saliva. Because people with AIDS have, in the past, donated blood which was used to make products for haemophiliacs, this group became the second largest group to have a high risk of AIDS. Some women develop AIDS through artificial insemination with infected semen. The third group to have a high risk of AIDS are intravenous drug-users. This is because unsterilised needles are generally used.

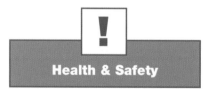

Health & Safety

Always use disposable equipment for ear-piercing and electrolysis to avoid the risk of transferring infection.

What does this mean to the hairdresser?

You are only at risk if blood is produced on cutting a client who has the AIDS virus (referred to as being HIV positive). As more people develop the virus, the risks will become greater. In salons, ear-piercing devices and electrolysis equipment present a possible route for transmitting the virus. You can protect yourself and the client by always covering cuts. If the skin has eczema, do not allow blood to come in contact under any circumstances. If blood is spilt in the salon it should be cleaned with household bleach, wearing gloves.

You can catch AIDS by:

Name	Appearance	Site of infection	Treatment
Herpes simplex – cold sore, a viral infection of the skin, it is believed to be triggered by ultraviolet light	A burning, prickly sensation followed by blisters filled with pus which develops into a dry crust	Lip, inside mouth and surrounding areas	Medical attention or pharmacist
Herpes zoster – shingles, a viral infection of the epidermis and nerve endings	Blisters appear, becoming inflamed and painful; symptoms are sometimes accompanied by a fever	Any part of the body	Medical attention
Warts, a viral infection of the skin	Raised rough skin, brown or discoloured	Fingers and hands, face and body, soles of feet	Medical attention

- having unprotected sex with someone who has the virus
- having infected blood enter a break in your skin
- infection by ear-piercing or electrolysis equipment
- infected blood coming in contact with skin with eczema
- sharing of needles if you are a drug user
- blood transfusion – however, all blood is now screened for the virus before use
- use of unsterilised or inadequately sterilised equipment.

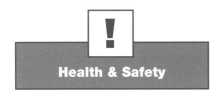

Health & Safety

Always wash hands thoroughly with anti-bacterial soap before and after every consultation.

Hepatitis B

Hepatitis B virus (HBV) is found in human blood and semen, and in contaminated water. The virus infects the liver causing weakness, and can be terminal. The treatment of hepatitis B, once diagnosed, is normally very successful. However, the virus is able to live outside the body therefore adequate hygiene is very important. Tools and equipment must be sterilised and disinfected regularly.

Hair loss

Alopecia

This is a general term meaning **baldness**. It may occur for a number of reasons which, as yet, are not fully understood.

The condition can be either permanent or temporary. Although alopecia is a general term, a number of specific kinds can be differentiated. So much psychological significance is attached to the possession of a head of luxuriant hair that a complaint of thinning hair is a frequent one, even if the individual is losing only the normal average of 60–100 hairs per day.

To determine whether the complaint of hair loss is genuine, an individual should be asked to collect and count hairs lost on the comb the day before washing, after washing and in the two succeeding days – four days in all. An average daily loss of over 100 hairs is abnormally high.

Hair loss can be divided into acute hair fall and a gradual loss which leads to a pattern of baldness. The table summarises types of hair loss, some of which are described in detail below.

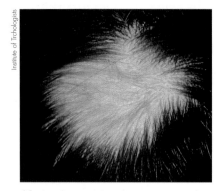

Alopecia areata

Alopecia areata

This is the most common type of acute hair loss. It is characterised by a loss of hair in round or oval, well-defined patches, without inflammation. The cause is not known and both sexes are equally affected. It is most common during childhood, although any age may be affected. In some instances the cause may be hereditary (about 20% of cases). Many cases have psychological factors associated with them and although this is perhaps the major cause associated with the condition, there are also many cases with no apparent emotional condition.

Onset of the condition is usually sudden, sometimes overnight. The size of the area involved varies from the size of a small coin to palm size or larger. The scalp is soft and smooth. At the sides of the spreading bald patches, exclamation hairs are present (!). These strands of hair are thicker at the ends and taper towards the root. When the exclamation hairs disappear, balding has been arrested and regrowth may not be certain but is usual.

The first hairs to reappear are white, soft and downy. These are soon replaced by thicker ones which give a piebald appearance. These are replaced by normal pigmented hairs.

With repeated attacks of hair loss, the chances of regrowth are lessened. Recovery is usual within 3–6 months of loss and no treatment is necessary when the individual is reassured, although a harmless local placebo may be given.

● **Alopecia totalis:** This term refers to complete loss of scalp hair – the eyebrows and eyelashes may also be involved.

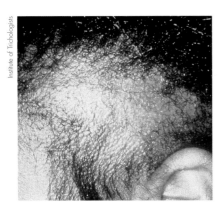

Traction alopecia

- **Alopecia universalis:** This is the term used for complete loss of hair from the body.

- **Alopecia senilis:** This is the thinning of the hair associated with old age. It does not always occur and can be caused by inadequate nutrition to the hair follicles.

- **Traction alopecia:** This is caused by harsh treatment of the hair by the individual. The bald patches are apparent at the crown or at the hairline. The cause may be overuse of a harsh brush, the strain of a pony tail, the strain of tightly wound rollers or pins or more commonly when braiding is too tight.

- **Cicatrical alopecia:** This is caused by chemical (relaxer) or physical (hot comb pressing) scarring after injury. Damage is caused to the hair follicles. This alopecia is irreversible, with the skin in the affected area remaining smooth, shiny and devoid of hair.

- **Diffuse alopecia:** This is apparent as constant daily hair loss over and above the normal level, from all areas of the scalp. The hair may eventually become very thin.

Male pattern baldness

The loss of hair on the frontal region and over the vertex may begin soon after puberty in males. There is a strong genetic factor involved. The male hormones, the androgens, appear to have an associated effect on this type of alopecia. Besides grafting follicles from the occipital region of the scalp to the bald areas, or applying female hormone (bringing associated undesirable side-effects) there are no remedies.

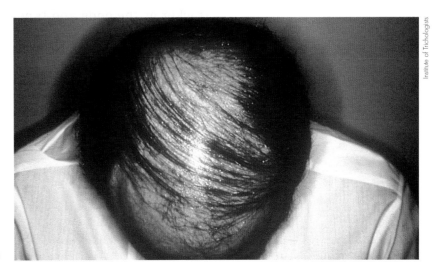

Male pattern baldness

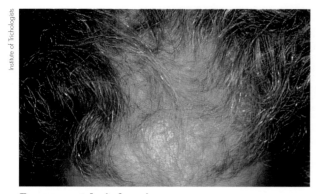

Permanent hair loss in women

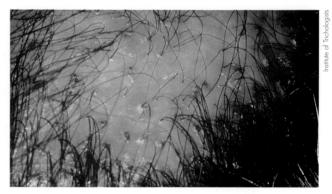

Hair loss in women

Thinning of the scalp hair over the vertex and top of the head is common in menopausal women and there may be marked baldness in extreme old age. Very rarely, thyroidism may be the cause of hair loss. The hair loss is similar to male hair loss and may also have a strong genetic factor. Usually the hair loss is only partial. Diffuse alopecia may occur in young women as a result of using oral contraceptives. It may last from several months to 2 years.

Hirsuties

Hirsuties is also known by the term hypertrichosis or excessive hair and is usually hereditary. It signifies superfluous hair and is found on areas which would naturally have downy hair (arms, face, etc.). Although it occurs in both men and women, it is usually only a distressing complaint in women. The majority of women who suffer from overgrowth of facial hair do not suffer from any demonstrable disorders and the trait is often due to hormones, use of medication, or shock.

Electrolysis can be used to remove facial hair permanently. This should only be carried out by a trained electrologist. The hair can also be bleached so that it is less noticeable.

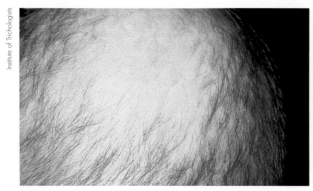

Diffuse hair loss

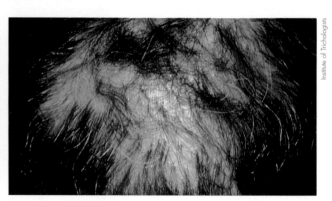

Cicatrical alopecia

Types of hair loss

Disorder	Definition	Location	Cause	Signs	Treatment
Alopecia	Baldness or thinning of hair	Anywhere on the scalp, usually the crown	Unsure, however, could be hereditary, caused by stress and/or psychological	Increase in daily hair loss totally or locally	See a trichologist or seek medical attention
Alopecia areata	Round bald patches on scalp seen often in hairdressing	Anywhere on the scalp	Unsure, however, could be hereditary, caused by stress and/or psychological	Small to large bald patch	As above
Alopecia totalis	Progressive alopecia areata resulting in total loss of scalp hair	Scalp hair, eyebrows, eyelashes	Can be caused by shock/trauma		As above
Alopecia universalis	Complete loss of body hair; a very rare condition	All over the body	The hair follicle cannot replace old hair with new		As above
Traction alopecia	Hair loss due to traction	Crown and hairline	Constant pulling of the hair shaft, for example pony tails, braids, hairpieces, hot combing	Thinning of hair in crown or hairline region; sore, tender scalp	See a trichologist
Cicatrical alopecia	Hair loss due to scarred tissue	Anywhere on the scalp	Physical or chemical damage due to scalp injury; damage to hair follicle is permanent	Sore tender scalp; result after chemical burns	See a trichologist
Post-partum alopecia	Hair loss after pregnancy	Mainly crown, but can be any area on the scalp	Reduced levels of hormone production after birth of child	Increased hair fall	Seek medical advice
Male pattern baldness	Baldness found in younger men and older women	Front, top and crown on scalp	Hereditary	Thinning of the hair in crown or centre of head	Hair transplant
Diffuse hair loss	General thinning of the hair	All over the head	Changes in hormonal level, pregnancy, contraceptive pill, illness, diabetes, fever and anaemia	Hair loss exceeding 100 hairs per day; the old hair is not replaced by new ones	See a trichologist

Animal parasites

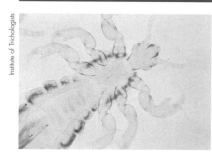

Head louse

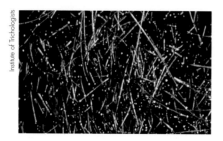

Head lice

A parasite lives in or on a living organism and causes it harm. If it lives outside the body it is called an **ecto-parasite**. If it lives inside the body it is known as an **endo-parasite**.

Pediculosis – lice

There are three types of lice, named according to the parts of the body they infest:

- Pediculus capitis – head
- Pediculus pubis – pubic area
- Pediculus corporis – body

Scabies

Scabies is caused by an allergic reaction to a mite. This and other common animal parasites are described in the table.

Animal parasites

Disease	Definition	Location	Cause	Signs	Transmission	Treatment
Pediculosis capitis, head lice	An infestation of the head by lice	Head – normally in the occipital region	The louse pierces the host to feed on blood	Profound itching and irritation accompanied by tiny red spots in the contaminated area	Direct contact	Seek medical attention or consult pharmacist
Pediculosis pubis, pubic lice	An infestation of the pubic hair by lice	Mainly the pubic region, but could be found anywhere on the body	As above	As above	Direct contact	Seek medical attention
Pediculosis corporis, body lice	An infestation of the clothing with lice which is then transferred to the body	Anywhere on the body	As above	As above	Direct contact	Seek medical attention
Scabies	An allergic reaction to an itch mite, *Sarcoptes scabei*	Wherever the skin folds or wrinkles, i.e. inbetween the fingers, the wrists and elbows	The mite burrows through the skin	Long, red lines in the skin covered with small lumps or blisters; severe itching at night when the skin is moist	Indirect or direct contact	Seek medical attention

Index